Girth Matters

A Comprehensive Guide to Nonsurgical Male Enhancement.

Luis Casavantes, MD

FOREWORD

This book describes for the first time the currently safest technique of penis enlargement. Based on his years of experience with thousands of patients, Dr. Casavantes has succeeded in creating an entertaining, sometimes humorous, and, above all, never boring work. All chapters are illustrated with comprehensible pictures, which facilitate reading and understanding.

There is no better way to educate doctors and laymen simultaneously about the anatomy and function of the penis, the simple but very well thought-out technique of the problematic penis enlargement, and the mention of all possible complications are impressively described by the world's foremost expert. And the last chapter, with some typical anecdotes from the life of a penis expert, adds a bit of humor to such a serious topic. Unfortunately, many men get in their own way when it comes to penis enlargement, so the enlarger must be a good psychologist at the same time.

In addition, Dr. Casavantes mentions all alternative possibilities of penis enlargement with the necessary criticism of the expert and openly describes the psychological backgrounds of his patients, which are mainly based on a misunderstood self-esteem. The majority have an average-sized penis but have been made insecure by porn actors and false ads and think much too critically about their best piece.

Women usually don't care about the length of a penis, but some may wish for a thicker penis. What men, however, often don't want to take to heart is that even during the sexual act, women are mainly concerned with tenderness, empathy, and proof of love.

Thousands of men have regained their self-confidence through the injections of Dr. Casavantes, and thousands of men will continue to be grateful to him for perfecting his technique. It is also possible that one or two will be moved to reconsider their desire for augmentation after reading this enlightening book.

Gottfried Lemperle, MD, PhD
Division of Plastic Surgery
University of California, San Diego

ABOUT THE AUTHOR

Luis Casavantes never intended to become a dick doctor. His story begins on a ranch in the idyllic countryside of Chihuahua. He had a bike, a horse, a dog, and no need for anything more.

His ambition was to go to university to become a doctor, but he didn't immediately know what branch of medicine to focus on. By his own admission, Casavantes went through everything in medical school. He started out studying neurology, but soon realized that most of his patients would end up dying or paralyzed, and he knew he couldn't personally handle that. He then moved on to cardiology, but found it uninspiring, and listening to the sound of blood pumping through hearts right after lunch made him queasy. Then early one morning while pacing the university campus a thought struck him that changed the trajectory of his life: why not dermatology? Casavantes suddenly realized that for some reason he loved dermatology, and he immediately enrolled at the top school in the country for the the discipline and began studying under Mexico's first dermatologist.

His timing couldn't have been more perfect. By the time Dr. Casavantes graduated, a global revolution in dermatology was underway. This was the start of botox, lasers, and fillers; the beginning of dermatology moving away from just being about acne and skin cancer to embracing advanced cosmetic procedures that were changing people's appearances and, by extension, their lives. The young Casavantes jumped right into the fray, learned how to use many different types of fillers and began injecting cheeks, lips, and other areas of the face.

Then one day in 2002, Luis Casavantes's path took a dramatic turn. A young man walked into his office who was looking prematurely aged. His face was sunken in; he looked almost skeletal. Casavantes injected some hyaluronic acid to rebuild his cheeks, and when he was finished he handed the patient a mirror. When he saw himself he began crying tears of joy. While the doctor welcomed this reaction, he did not yet fully understand it — he was like "what did I do?"

Soon after that patient left another walked in who had a similar condition — young male, prematurely aging — looking for facial fillers, then another, then another, then another. Word was spreading as to what Dr. Casavantes could do, and his schedule was soon fully booked with this type of patient. He realized that this couldn't have been coincidental, so he did a little research and discovered who these young me were: HIV patients who were experiencing facial lipoatrophy as a result of their medication.

While hyaluronic acid was a quick fix for these patients, the results were temporary, often only lasting around six months. Casavantes knew that this was not sustainable — they needed a permanent solution. Many of these men were hiding from society, embarrassed about their appearance, fearful of the stigma attached to their condition. So he began scouring the world for a filler that wouldn't dissolve and go away, and after a few dead ends found what he was looking for in Brazil: Polymethyl methacrylate, most commonly known as PMMA. Casavantes was now able to restore the faces of patients with HIV-related lipoatrophy to normalcy, permanently, enabling them to return to their lives.

At this time there was only a few doctors in the world doing this type of procedure for these patients, and Dr. Casavantes's office became inundated with them. He worked seven days a week but didn't care — the work gave him a sense of purpose that mere beautification procedures never could. He felt as if he was giving his patients their lives back.

But fate would again intervene, as one of his facial hypotrophy patients one day asked if he was able to inject PMMA in his penis. "If you could do a face why can't you do a penis?" the patient reasoned — a statement that Casavantes could not argue with. So he tried it, injecting the filler into the areolar space of the patient's penis in hopes that it would increase its girth. Almost to their surprise the results were outstanding.

Then it happened again. That first girth enhancement patient referred another, who referred another, who referred another. Word of mouth transitioned to online postings on penis enlargement forums like Phalloboards, and before long men looking for thicker penises began flocking to Tijuana to see Casavantes, who eventually became better known as Dr. C, the world's preeminent dick doctor.

* * *

The timing couldn't have been more perfect, as advances in HIV medication did away with the lipoatrophy side effect, and transitioning to penises allowed Dr. C to continue doing what he found most satisfying: giving men the confidence to go out and live their lives to the fullest. "Small penis syndrome" impacts nearly half of all men — some of them so severely that they avoid dating or engaging in sexual activity. Like sufferers of HIV-induced facial hypotrophy, some of these men are in hiding, too embarrassed to fully engage the world around them, living in fear that someone will discover their condition.

Early on, Dr. C found that his non-surgical girth enhancement treatment was effective at combating "small penis syndrome," and over the next 15 years perfected his methods, performing the procedure on over 4,000 men from all over the world. In a frontier of medicine that often attracts unscrupulous "doctors" who do shoddy treatments with untested products, Dr. C was a beacon of best practices and professionalism, almost singlehandedly transforming the reputation of phalloplasty for the good and reducing risks down below that of breast augmentation. His 90% satisfaction rate speaks for itself, as does the fact that over 60% of his patients return for more.

Now Dr. C is on the verge of retirement, having gained worldwide recognition for his work, and is passing the torch on to Dr. Morales and his staff at his clinic, Avanti Derma. The only thing that is still needed for him to complete his journey is a little house at the end of the road somewhere beautiful.

CHAPTER ONE

A Brief History of Penis Enhancement

Attempts to enlarge the male genitalia date back to the dawn of human history and span cultures throughout the world. From South America to Africa to Asia, men have attempted to increase the size of their penises via stretching, herbs, and, for the Tupinambá people of Brazil at least, the bite of a poisonous snake. The quest for a larger penis has seemingly always been an obsession of the human male.

The first incidences of effective surgical intervention by qualified physicians were described in 1971 by Kelley and Eraklis [1], who published a successful method for penile elongation in children with specific birth defects.

As for girth enhancement, which is the topic of this book, we had to wait a further decade for a Miami-based surgeon, Dr. Samiter, to introduce his new procedure. However, his 'innovation' was more of a new application for autologous fat transfer, an existing surgical technique consisting of taking fat from one part of the body and moving it to another. In theory, it was a relatively straightforward procedure, by which a small amount of fat is harvested by liposuction, usually from the abdomen or inner thigh area, and then injected under the skin of the penis to add thickness. Initially, things looked good — the procedure could be completed in under one hour and offered substantial gains in girth along with supposedly minimal side effects.

Unsurprisingly, autologous fat transfer proved to be a popular method, which was soon adopted by many other surgeons. Eventually, demand was so high that some clinicians were performing as many as ten per day. However, as so often is the case, not all that glitters is gold: it soon became apparent that there were drawbacks that often had devastating consequences for the men who had undergone this procedure. Patients started returning to those doctors so that they could reverse their undesirable results or get reconstructive surgeries to repair the damage.

Autologous fat transfer's critical deficiencies were primarily related to irregularities resulting from the limited vascular uptake of the transferred fat [2]. Unfortunately, between 10% and 90% of the injected fat is reabsorbed unevenly in the months following surgery, leaving the penis with an irregular contour. The remaining fat tends to form palpable fatty cysts or solid nodules, creating lumps and other defects. An added issue was the fact that free fat lacks the necessary rigidity to feel natural when the penis is in the erect state. Needless to say, a penis that both looked and felt unnatural simply was not desirable for most men.

* * *

However, the demand for a perfect image and the feeling of being more prominent and impressive was so high that surgeons kept looking for alternatives to enhance the size of the human penis. The next attempt came from California, where Los Angeles based surgeons, such as Dr. Alter and Dr. Rheinschild, pioneered a method of increasing girth with dermal fat grafts [3].

While this method also transplanted tissue under the skin of the penis, the fundamental differences between free fat transfer and dermal fat grafts is that the former is free fat obtained through liposuction and the latter consists of blocks or strips of subcutaneous tissue cut through surgery, usually from the gluteal crease or the lower abdomen. Chances of graft survival increased by keeping the fat intact and attached to the dermis and its blood vessels without going through the physically exhausting and demanding liposuction process. The procedure required incisions at the neck of the penis to position the strips of fat and dermis under the skin and stitches to anchor them at both ends.

The dermal graft technique improved significantly and resulted in fewer and smaller irregularities and tended to be smoother and less palpable, while gains were usually more generous. However, these benefits came at a cost, as it soon became apparent that dermal grafts had their own set of drawbacks and complications.

* * *

The first set of issues derived from the surgical process itself, which is highly invasive compared to the free fat transfer method. It takes several hours to perform and requires an arduous recovery. While free fat transfers are virtually scar-free, dermal grafting resulted in extensive and often unsightly donor and entry site scarring. The long incisions, particularly those made in the gluteal creases and pubic area, required drains and stitches and had a high risk of infection.

The second group of issues was related to how the grafts themselves behaved after their insertion. Though the surgeon would suture them into place, the grafts were never genuinely secure until vascular blood supply took place. Moving and twisting of the graft during the recovery period resulted in deformities and retraction of the penis. Perhaps the most significant enemies of dermal grafts were contracture and tissue necrosis. Often times during the weeks following surgery the grafts would shrink, leaving areas filled with fibrotic material and an excess of hard tissue associated with the reparative or reactive process. This fibrotic tissue made the grafts less pliable to the point that they would not sufficiently stretch to accommodate the length of the penis during an erection. In the end, the graft contracture could be severe, leaving the penis shorter or bent; also, if part of the graft failed to achieve sufficient blood supply, it would turn necrotic, die, and be reabsorbed, which again deformed both the look and touch of the penis.

* * *

Even though dermal grafts had some satisfying results, most surgeons felt that, due to high complication rates, the risks were too high, and very few adopted the method. Today, this method has become virtually obsolete.

The efforts to find better alternatives for girth enhancement continued; this time, the pendulum swung back to the east coast of the US, where a New York surgeon named Dr. Whitehead experimented with biomaterials, such as a regenerative tissue matrix derived from the skin of human cadavers called allografts.

Allografts are sheets of biological substance successfully used for hernia repair, dental procedures, and breast reconstruction. They bypass the need to harvest and prepare grafts from other parts of the patient's body, reduce surgery time, and avoid some of the incisions which often leave the patient with visible scars and deformities in the donor site. At the time, this became the preferred method of treatment for penile enlargement, even though it did come with certain drawbacks.

The grafts were expensive, and typically would only be about one-third as thick as a dermal fat graft, meaning that patients would be paying more but gaining significantly less size. Other than the benefits achieved by avoiding harvesting the tissue from the patient, the issues remained consistent with those reported with the dermal fat graft technique: contracture, hardening, necrosis, complete or partial absorption, slippage, and infection [4,5]. Hence, as with its predecessors, allografts have never been widely adopted for penis enlargement by the surgical community.

At the turn of the century, doctors kept experimenting with various other implant materials, such as pre-formed solid 'soft' silicone sheets or firm silicone and PLGA (Poly Lactide-co-Glycolide) scaffolds among others, but again with limited success. Surgeons have failed to find a consensus to support anyone's method, and penis enlargement remains a widely controversial subject, with only a small fraction of physicians prepared or willing to perform these surgeries.

Ultimately, the penis is a uniquely complex organ to augment due to its dynamic nature as well as its variations in size and consistency between its flaccid and erect states present the biggest challenge to find an appropriate implant material or method. The implant must be soft when flaccid, yet firm when erect; it should also be able to stretch sufficiently to accommodate erections and must not interfere with the process of urination and ejaculation.

So the medical community was left with only one conclusion to consider: Perhaps surgery is not the answer?

Nonsurgical Penile Girth Enhancement (Nonsurgical Phalloplasty)

* * *

The arrival of soft tissue fillers presented a genuine alternative for penile girth enhancement: a nonsurgical option that delivered the desired results with lower risks of complications.

Modern procedures moved away from aggressive surgical operations to in-office methods that required no hospitalization, general anesthesia, incisions, drains, stitches, scars, or prolonged downtime. When experienced physicians followed the proper injection techniques the most common complications were reduced to rare occurrences.

It is fair to conclude that nonsurgical cosmetic medicine started in the early ninety-eighties with the introduction of bovine collagen [6] as the first injectable filler designed to correct minor facial tissue deficits and imperfections or to enhance small areas like the lips.

Soon after the introduction of medical cosmetic products and procedures, dermatology practices started accepting healthy patients looking for non-invasive treatments that improved their looks and elevated their self-esteem. Before long, the list of soft tissue-based cosmetic treatments grew from correcting frown lines and crow's feet to complete facial reconstruction, hand rejuvenation, and penile girth enhancement [7], to mention a few.

* * *

This book covers the new trend of surgery-free, hospital-free penile girth enhancement (nonsurgical phalloplasty) with injectable soft tissue fillers, explaining the available procedures and products, expected results, and possible complications.

Readers are invited to visit the book's associated website, www.girthmatters.com. They can see an extended before & after photo gallery and find out about updates on girth enhancement procedures and soft tissue fillers.

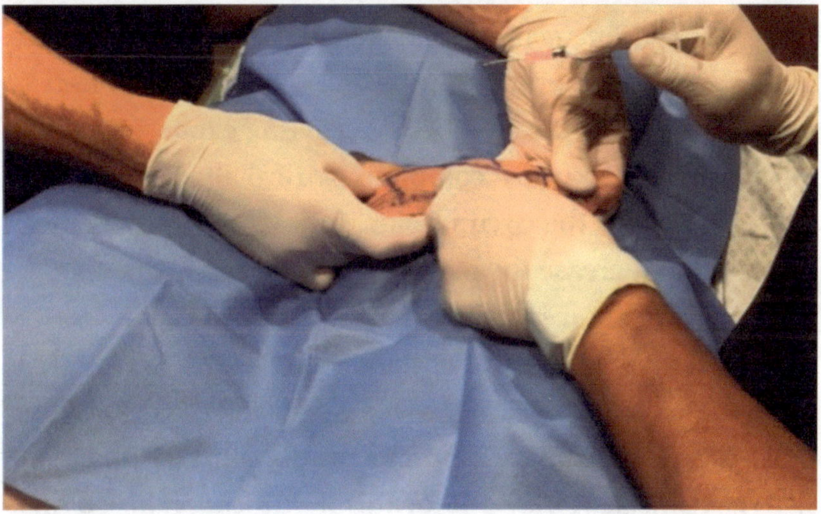

Figure 1.1. Nonsurgical phalloplasty using injection gun, micro cannulas, and permanent soft tissue filler Linnea Safe™.

CHAPTER TWO

Basic Concepts

Bodily modification, reconstruction, and mutilation dates back to prehistoric times and include physical changes mainly used to make facial structures, the neck, and genitalia more appealing to others or to better perceive themselves.

Penile elongation techniques have been a common practice in different ethnic groups, and they have done this often without the scientific knowledge of tissue expansion. In modern times, the most common medical alteration of male genitalia is the circumcision, followed by procedures designed to increase the length and, later on, the penis's width. A large percentage of male individuals have insecurities about the size of their penis, which is why they opt to have it enlarged. However, this is not the case with most people who go for genitalia mutilation, as is the case with circumcision they opt for this modification based on religious reasons or use the well-documented argument that the procedure creates a more hygienic way to live.

There is evidence that male genitalia mutilation originated in Africa, long before the biblical account of Abraham that ordered circumcision (Genesis 17:10-11): "This is my covenant with you and your descendants after you, the covenant you are to keep: Every male among you shall be circumcised. You are to undergo circumcision, and it will be the sign of the covenant between you and me."

The Jews adopted the ancient practice of circumcision as a religious ritual, and they have preserved it until modern times [8], in contrast to the Greeks and Romans who placed a high value on the foreskin to the extent of passing laws to protect it [9].

The lower third of the vagina houses the main nerve supply, and most women feel more excited when having it stretched to its optimal extent with a thicker penis rather than being penetrated deeply by a longer one. In other words, a thick penis seems to be a better male attribute.

Since a large percentage of men are not satisfied with the size of their penis, the demand to increase it is high and has led to many attempts at correction. Until a decade ago, most penile girth enhancement procedures relied on surgery, but complications like scarring, deformity, and necrosis were common. The arrival of injectable soft tissue fillers diminished the frequency and severity of the complications, offering a much safer alternative by moving towards non-invasive, in-office procedures that require no cuts, drains, stitches, permanent scars, or prolonged downtime.

Six by Six, or More!

* * *

A review of over 30 published medical research reports involving 15,521 men [10] has shown that the average size of the erect human penis is 13.12 cm (5.2") in length and 11.66 cm (4.6") in circumference. However, most men do not like the word average or standard when it comes to their penis size. Most prospective patients seeking to increase their penis' size hope to reach or surpass the ideal mark of 15 centimeters (6") in both length and circumference. For some, it is an ambitious goal, but many others who have achieved this 'ideal size' want even more. Patients in a heterosexual relationship tend to justify their desire for volume increase by claiming that it's to please their female partners, even though the latter typically have no complaints. On the other hand, the gay population is more likely to admit that they are doing the procedure to improve their self-esteem.

Scientific studies show that a majority of women find both length and girth to be unimportant [11]. However, this does not stop many men from wanting a massive penis, which they equate with sexual power, prowess, and masculinity.

Statistics

Research has shown that 45% of the male population is unhappy with their penis size. A report combining 50 studies and covering more than 11,000 individuals showed that 85% of women were satisfied with their partners' dimensions, while only 55% of the male counterparts felt they had measured up [12]. In an internet study of 52,031 people, 66% of participants rated their penis size as average, 22% as big, and 12% as small [13].

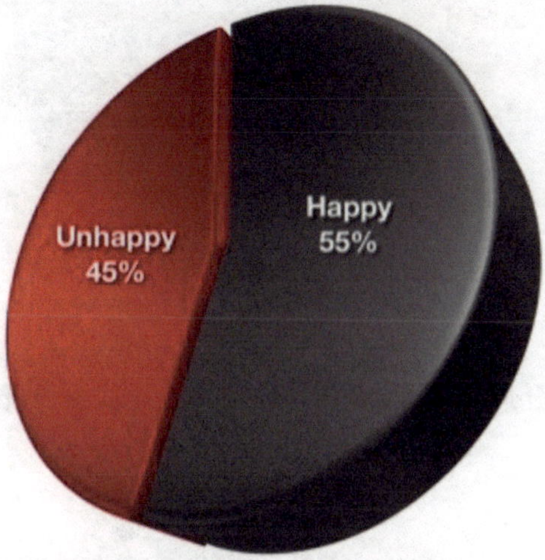

Figure 2.1. Men's satisfaction with the size of their penis.

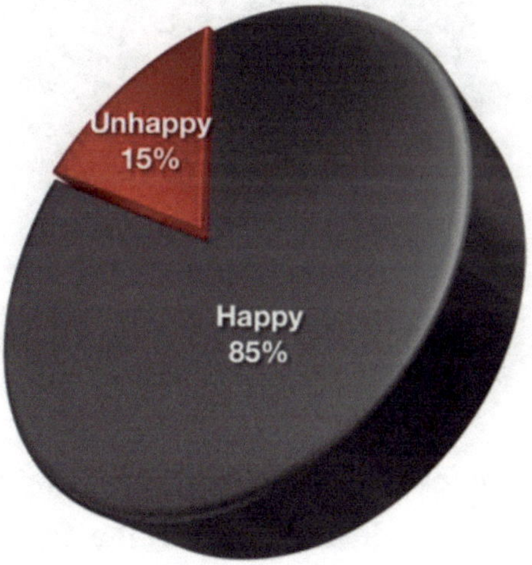

Figure 2.2. Women's satisfaction with the size of their partner's penis.

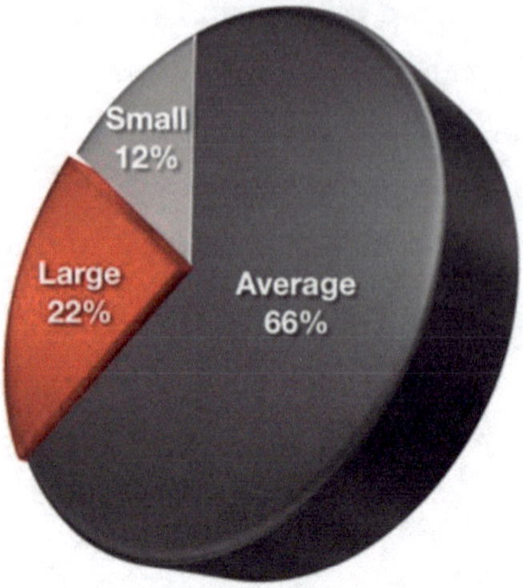

Figure 2.3. Men's self-evaluation of the size of their penis.

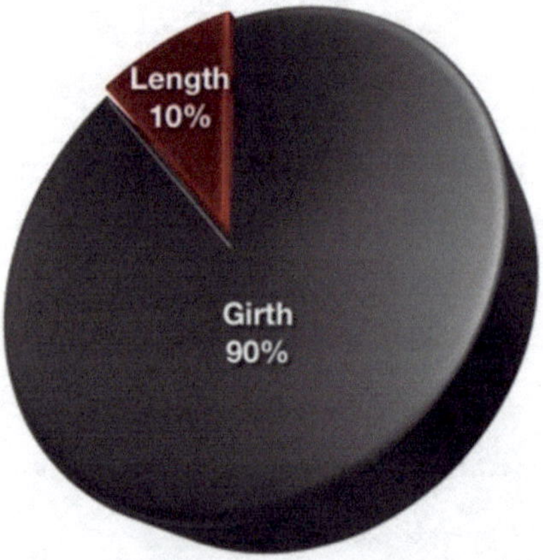

Figure 2.4. Woman's preference: girth vs. length.

As mentioned before, most data suggest that penis size is small on the list of male attributes that attract women to men. According to a study using 3D models, women preferred penises that were only slightly larger than average [14].

Available Techniques

The demand for male genitalia enhancement procedures has triggered the imagination of both researchers and practitioners. The list grows as new products (mainly soft tissue fillers) and methods become available.

Even though the injection techniques are similar, nonsurgical phalloplasty patients have the option to decide on temporary, long-lasting, or permanent alternatives.

<table>
<tr><th>Procedure</th><th>Surgical</th><th>Nonsurgical</th></tr>
<tr><td>Penile elongation</td><td>Suspensory ligament release
Scrotal webbing removal</td><td>Mechanical traction</td></tr>
<tr><td>Girth augmentation</td><td>Free fat transfer (FTT)
Dermal fat grafts
Scaffoldings
Soft silicone implants</td><td rowspan="3">Injectable
soft tissue fillers</td></tr>
<tr><td>Scrotal enhancement</td><td>Silicone prosthesis</td></tr>
<tr><td>Glans enhancement</td><td>-</td></tr>
</table>

Table 2.1. Male Genitalia Enhancement Procedures.

CHAPTER THREE

Male Genitalia

The best way to understand the nonsurgical penile girth enhancement procedures is to know the basic anatomy of the penis, scrotum, and other related body structures. The penis not only protrudes outside the body but also continues internally into the pelvis, all the way back to the prostate and pubic bones, almost reaching the rectum.

As shown below, the penis is divided into three main areas:

- **The radix (root):** The inner portion of the penis that is not visible. It sits on the pelvic cavity floor and extends from the back abdominal wall to the perineum (the erogenous zone between the testicles and the anus).
- **The body (shaft):** The continuation of the radix that extends outside the abdominal wall creating the visible part of the penis.
- **The glans**: The head of the penis.

* * *

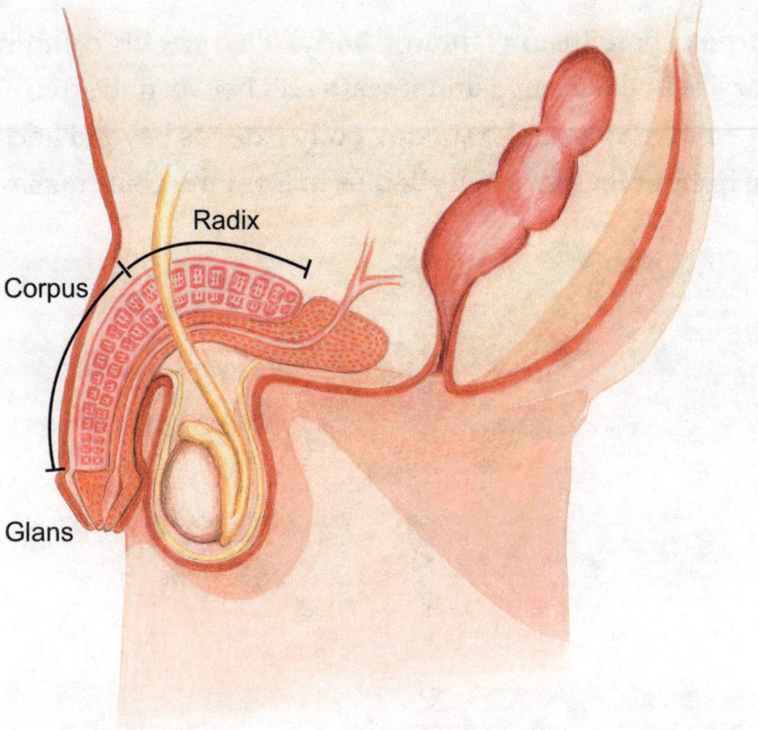

Figure 3.1. The three main divisions of the penis: Radix (root), Corpus (shaft), and glans.

The corpus penis is a single unit formed by the internal (radix) and external (body) segments of the penis. It houses three erectile organs that consist of columns of porous, expandable, sponge-like tissue:

Corpora cavernosa (cavernous bodies): Two erectile columns that lie next to each other on top of the corpus penis, which extend from the back of the glans to the radix, where they separate to form the crus (or crux) of the penis.

Corpus spongiosum (spongy body): One erectile column that lies in the groove underneath and between the two cavernous bodies. The spongy body extends beyond and to the front of the cavernous bodies to form the glans penis.

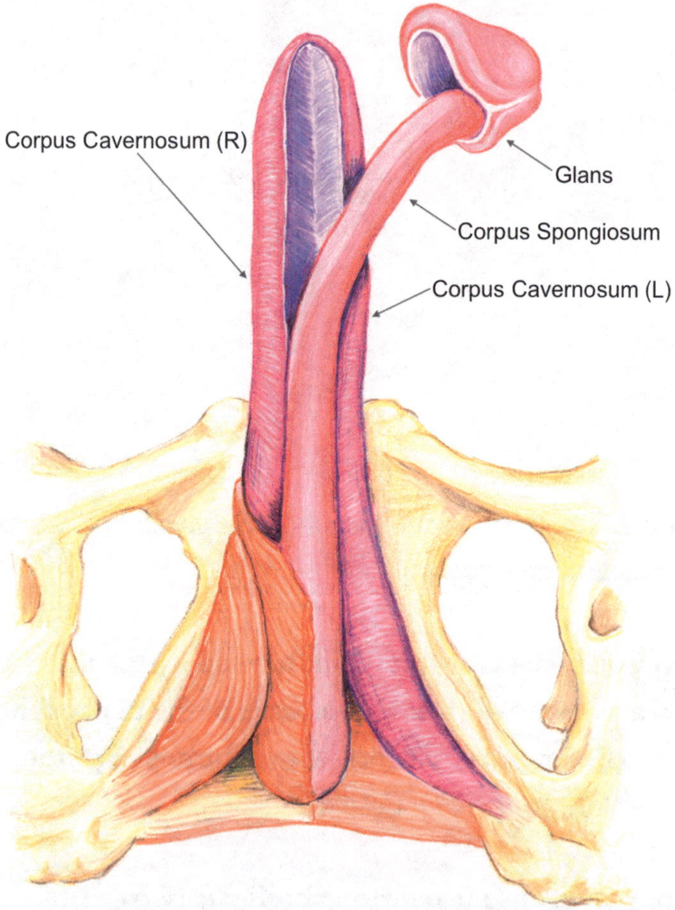

Figure 3.2. Erectile organs of the penis. Two cavernosum bodies and one spongy body which transforms into the glans at the end.

* * *

The urethra runs deep through the length of the corpus spongiosum and opens up at the tip of the glans penis in a vertical slit known as the urinary meatus.

In a transversal section view (Figure 3.3), the cavernous bodies are the two large formations (purple) that lie next to each other in the top portion, forming the bulk of the penis. Note the vast amount of cavernous and spongy areas that give these structures their name.

The cavernosal arteries run through the center of each cavernous body and are the principal blood supply that fills this tissue during an erection.

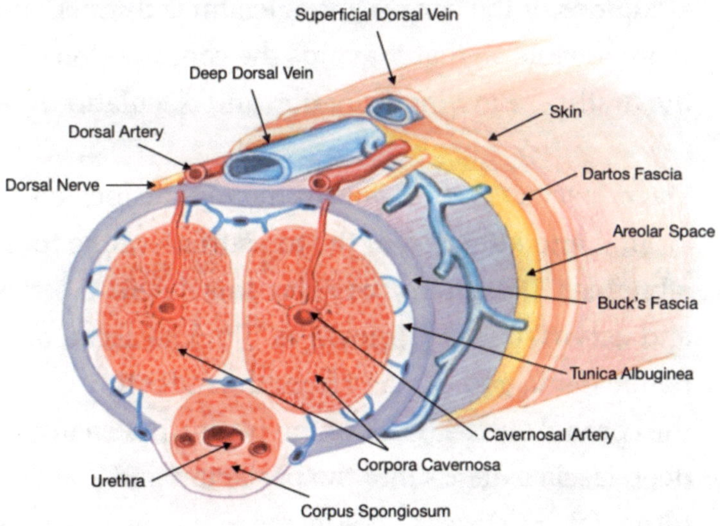

Figure 3.3. Transversal section of the penis.

* * *

Several layers of soft tissue surround the three erectile cylinders and bind them together. Knowing these layers is essential to understand the penile girth enhancement procedures. Please refer to Figure 3.3 for the descriptions below, starting from the inner-depth to the surface of the penis:

- **Tunica albuginea:** A dense and fibrous membrane that encases both the corpora cavernosa and the corpus spongiosum. When the three erectile bodies swell during sexual arousal, pressure against the not-so-flexible tunica albuginea compresses nearby veins preventing blood from draining away; this phenomenon maintains the erection. The tunica albuginea of the corpus spongiosum is thinner and more flexible so that it avoids the compression of the urethra, allowing urination and ejaculation.

- **Deep fascia:** Another fibrous membrane located around and adhering to the top surface of the tunica albuginea. It contains the deep dorsal vein, arteries, and nerves. It is also known as "Buck's Fascia" or penile fascia and extends from the radix to the coronal sulcus (neck of the penis). Internally, the deep fascia extends into the perineum and ultimately encloses and adheres to the deep penile structures of the pubis and the urogenital diaphragm.

* * *

- **Areolar tissue:** This is a layer of loose connective tissue that's soft and elastic enough to allow the overlying tissues some movement. The areolar tissue (or areolar space) lays between the two fasciae of the penis and is where soft tissue fillers are injected.

- **Superficial fascia:** Also known as the dartos fascia or subcutaneous connective tissue, the superficial fascia is located on top of the areolar tissue. It is softer and thinner than the deep fascia. The superficial dorsal vein and the two superficial lateral veins run through this layer on the dorsal side of the penis. The superficial fascia contains abundant smooth muscle fibers and attaches loosely to the skin on top and to the deep fascia underneath.

- **Skin:** The external layer of the penis that protects the rest of the structures and extends forward to create the prepuce (foreskin) that covers the glans in uncircumcised individuals. The dartos fascia and the skin loosely stick to each other.

The structures mentioned above can be grouped into two primary bundles that surround the erectile organs:

- One thick, robust bundle formed by the tunica albuginea and the deep fascia.
- One superficial, softer bundle formed by the

superficial fascia and the skin.

Both bundles are separated by the areolar space, which is the injection site of soft tissue fillers. The areolar space runs through the whole shaft of the penis and ultimately disappears as the superficial and deep fasciae interlace together at the coronal sulcus behind the glans.

This intricate crossing of the two fasciae varies between individuals and ultimately dictates how close to the glans a soft tissue filler can be injected. The volume of injectable fillers depends on the room available in the areolar space through the length of the penis.

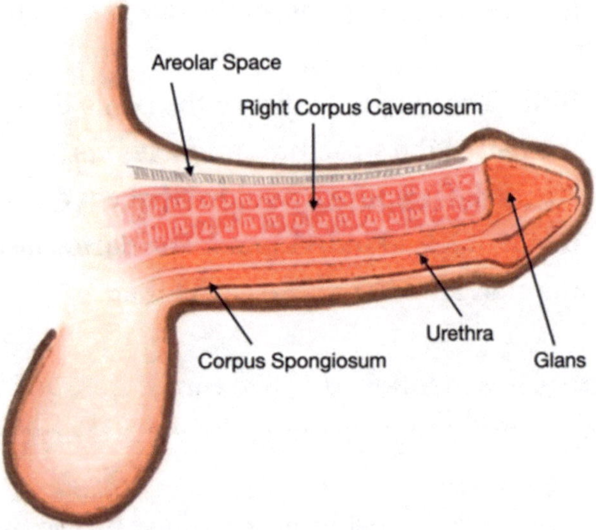

Figure 3.4. Longitudinal section of the penis showing the areolar

space.

A remarkable difference between the skin of the body and face compared to the penis is that the latter does not have any fat tissue underneath. When injectable soft tissue fillers are used in the face or anywhere else in the body, the subcutaneous fat tissue forms a soft cushion that can help camouflage imperfections, and the results are smooth and undetectable in most cases. Subcutaneous implants easily show under the skin of the penis.

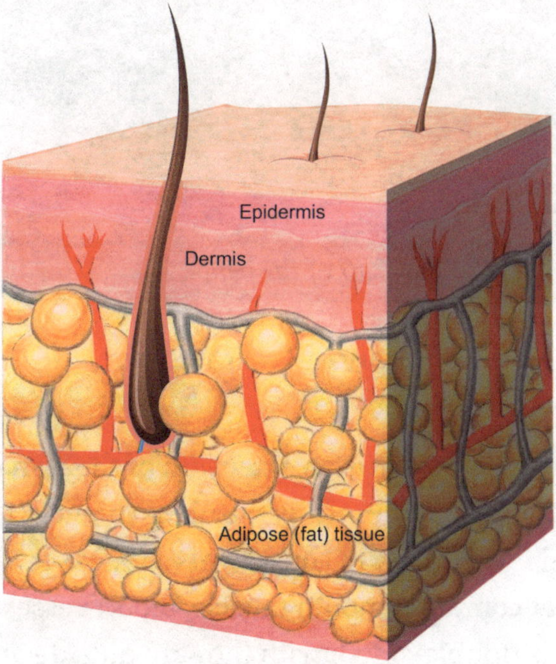

Figure 3.5. Skin of the face and body.

The skin over the fat-free penile tissues is thin, and soft

tissue fillers injected into the areolar space between the two fasciae are easily palpable and visible.

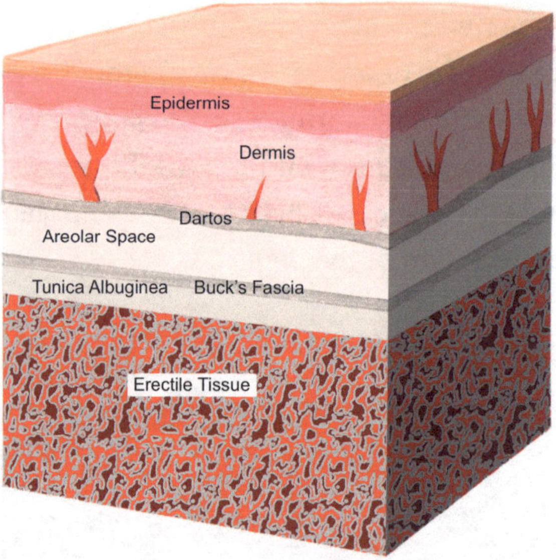

Figure 3.6. Skin of the shaft of the penis.

Prepuce: The foreskin

The prepuce (foreskin) is an extension of the skin of the penis that covers and protects the glans in uncircumcised individuals. The foreskin consists of a double-layered fold of skin that contains smooth muscle, blood vessels, and nerves. It is double-sided, with the skin outside and mucous membrane inside. It covers and protects the sensitive glans and the urinary meatus. The penile skin and prepuce create an oversized tissue envelope covering the penis, which stretches during erection and loosens when the penis is relaxed.

The relaxed, movable, and unsteady nature of the penile skin in the uncircumcised individual is one of the main challenges to maintain injectable fillers in their place of injection. In contrast, circumcised men have a more steady, almost non-movable, and less redundant skin that firmly covers the penis and facilitates the fillers' stability.

The foreskin covers the entire glans when the penis is at rest and can be retracted manually or spontaneously during erection. However, there are two pathological conditions in which the foreskin does not move freely:

Phimosis: When patients cannot fully retract their foreskin, leaving the glans partially covered at all times.

Paraphimosis: When the foreskin retracts but cannot be re-extended, leaving the glans unprotected.

The foreskin must remain intact after the injection of soft tissue fillers to preserve its flexibility and potential to retract and extend.

Circumcision

Circumcision is the surgical removal of the foreskin. It is a fairly standard procedure mainly performed on newborns in some parts of the world, including the United States. Different surgical techniques give different results; however, not all types of circumcision are ideal for phalloplasty patients.

We will discuss a classification that divides circumcision into four variants, according to the height of the scar and the skin's firmness.

Distal and tight

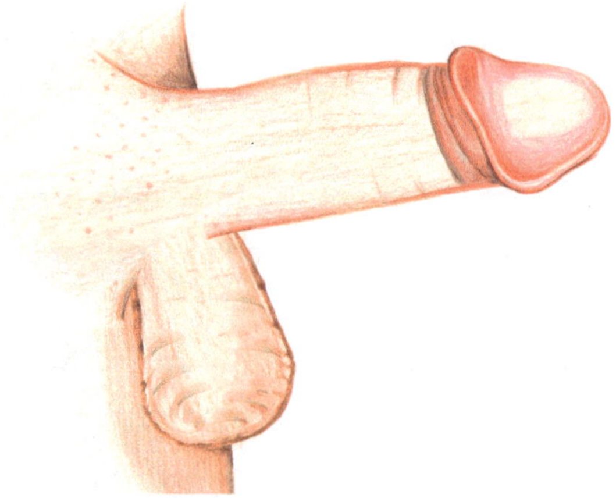

Figure 3.7. Distal and tight circumcision.

Colloquially known as "low and tight," this is the ideal circumcision variety for the nonsurgical phalloplasty patient.

"Distal" means that the circumcision scar locates near the neck of the penis (or the crown of the glans), leaving most of the shaft of the penis covered with its normal outer skin and minimally with remnants of the inner skin of the foreskin. In this way, the areolar space extends to the vicinity of the neck of the penis, and the soft tissue filler implant will reach that area.

"Tight" means that the skin is smooth, tense, and firm, which helps the soft tissue filler to remain in place, avoiding migration and shifting.

Proximal and tight

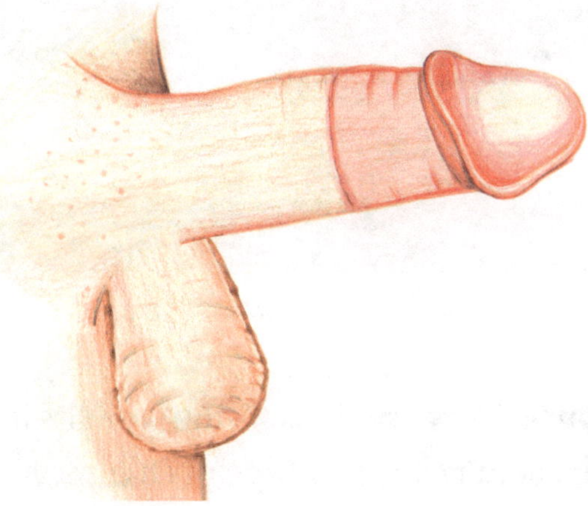

Figure 3.8. Proximal and tight circumcision.

Also known as "high and tight," the scar is located more towards the middle of the shaft, and the penis shows two types of skin: external in the proximal part and soft and pink (inner skin of the foreskin) in its distal portion. This type of circumcision distorts and shortens the areolar space, and the circumcision scar in the center of the shaft can create a compressive ring-shaped indentation that deforms the implant.

Distal and loose

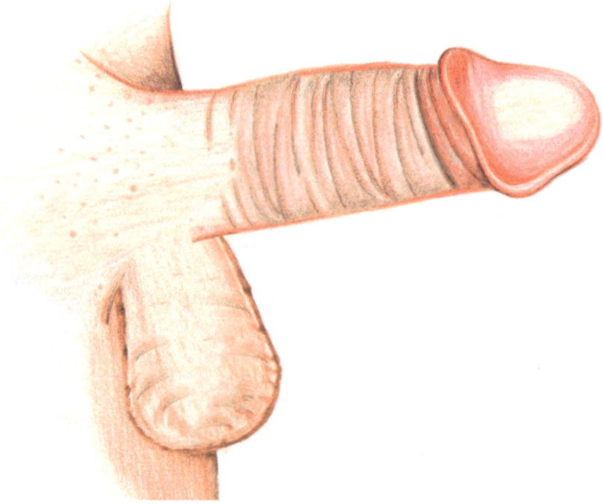

Figure 3.9. Distal and loose circumcision.

Also known as "low and loose," the scar sits in the correct area, but the skin is lax; this type of circumcision does not help hold the implant in place, and it can easily clump, migrate, or shift. These patients require using a compression bandage for several weeks, and it is better to use a low volume of soft tissue filler to avoid significant irregularities. High volume use in this type of patient can cause the unwanted effect known as "pig in a blanket." See the chapter on limitations and complications for more about this condition.

Proximal and loose

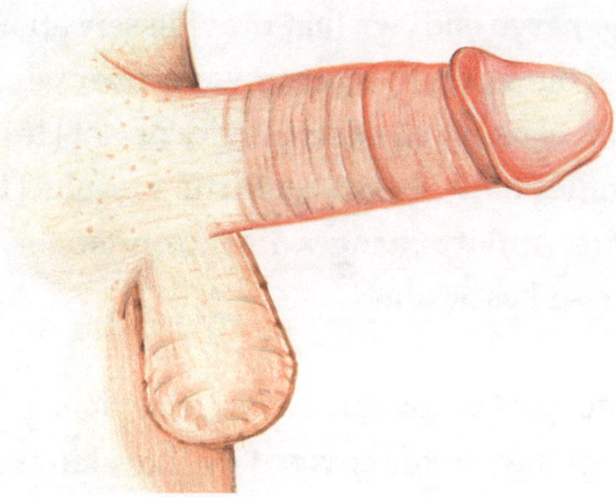

Figure 3.10. Proximal and loose circumcision.

Also known as "high and loose," it behaves like the "low and loose" variety, with the aggravation of the circumcision scar sitting in the middle of the shaft, which can create two separate implants with a constricting ring that also divides the two different skin types present in these patients.

Glans

The glans penis (or head of the penis) is the sensitive extension of the corpus spongiosum found at the end of the two corpora cavernosa. Its back surface has a crest called the corona (coronal sulcus), which drops backward to form the neck of the penis.

* * *

The sebaceous glands of the foreskin keep the glans moist, and the surgical removal of the foreskin (circumcision) exposes the glans permanently, turning the mucous membrane into slightly rough, dry skin. Since the glans contain free nerve endings that provide sensation during sexual intercourse, there is controversy over whether circumcision causes loss of sensitivity or not [15]. Clinical studies have shown conflicting results [16], but it seems that sensitivity changes are uncommon in men who are circumcised as adults.

At a microscopic (histological) level, the glans penis consists of spongy tissue covered by thin skin (squamous epithelium).

* * *

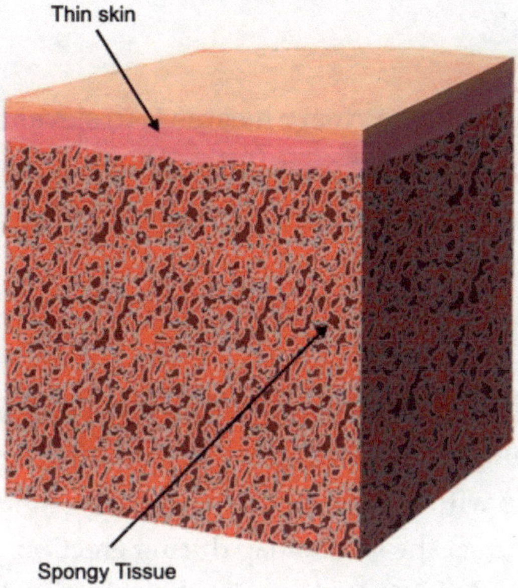

Figure 3.11. The thin skin of the glans.

Unlike the skin of the body, which has a thick layer of subcutaneous fat tissue, or the penis's skin with the areolar space, the glans has minimal room for injectable fillers.

The skin covering the glans is so thin that injectable soft tissue fillers can only be used in minimal amounts before they go directly into the bloodstream, collapses the local spongiosum tissue, or cause necrosis by compression.

The urinary meatus is the orifice at the end of the glans, where urine and semen come out. Although it typically opens at the tip of the glans, the meatus sometimes presents at a lower or higher exit point, creating malformations known as "hypospadias" and "epispadias," respectively.

The location of the urinary meatus is irrelevant in regards to the injection of soft tissue fillers, and it doesn't affect the eligibility of patients.

Scrotum and testicles

The scrotum is a dual-chambered, suspended sack of skin that contains the testicles. Deep in its surface lays a membrane with involuntary muscle fibers (dartos muscle), which contract the scrotal bag during erection, cold weather, and alarm. It also protects and regulates the temperature of the testicles.

The cremaster is a second muscle that descends from the abdomen and surrounds the testicles and the spermatic cord. This muscle elevates the testes, thereby regulating their temperature.

The scrotal septum is a membrane that divides the scrotal bag into two different cavities and causes the visible longitudinal depression that runs front to back over the entire scrotum.

Each of the two scrotal cavities contains one testicle and its related structures:

* * *

- The external spermatic fascia;
- The epididymis;
- The vas deferent (ducts that carry sperm from the testes to the penis);
- Isolated genital hairs cover the scrotum after puberty.

Physiology

The following section discusses the primary functions of the penis and its possible interactions with the injectable soft tissue fillers that are used for girth enhancement.

Erection

Penile tumescence (erection) is the process through which the penis becomes enlarged and firm due to multiple factors associated with sexual stimulation which pushes blood and pressure-fills the three erectile organs. The liberation of nitric oxide in the small arteries and smooth muscle fibers inside the cavernous and spongy bodies triggers the erection. The arteries then dilate as the erectile structures fill with blood. Simultaneously, other involuntary muscles and the pressure on the tunica albuginea and Buck's fascia compress the deep dorsal vein of the penis, restricting the blood flow back into the body and maintaining the erection.

* * *

During an erection, the corpora cavernosa holds about 90% of the blood, while the corpus spongiosum holds the rest, giving fullness to the glans penis while protecting the urethra from collapsing. The structures encasing the erectile structures beyond the tunica albuginea (Buck's fascia, areolar tissue, dartos fascia and the skin) expand but do not influence the erection of the penis.

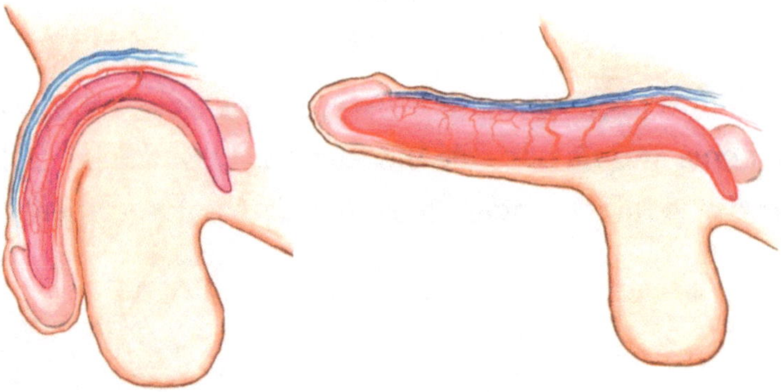

Figure 3.12. The penis in relaxation and erection.

It is essential to keep in mind that the entire penile erection process is triggered in the depth of the cavernous and spongy tissues, away from the area of injection of soft tissue fillers.

Erectile dysfunction

Erectile dysfunction refers to any condition that alters the course of an erection, and can range from impotence on one side of the spectrum to priapism (persistent and painful erection) on the other.

Impotence

Impotence is the inability to achieve or maintain an erection firm enough to engage in or finish sexual intercourse. It classifies as psychological and organic, but both factors can occur in the same individual.

The first one is mainly related to stress, and it only happens under certain circumstances; typically, it does not affect spontaneous or nocturnal arousals.

Organic impotence has specific underlying causes, such as medical conditions and the use of some medications, and it most likely affects nocturnal erections as well.

The following are the most common conditions associated with organic impotence:

- **Medical:** High blood pressure, arteriosclerosis, diabetes mellitus, chronic kidney or heart diseases, some tumors, anemia, and many others.
- **Medications:** Anti-hypertensive drugs, narcotics, estrogen, stimulants, psychotropic drugs, etc.
- **Lifestyle:** Alcohol, nicotine, antidepressants, caffeine, lack of sleep, etc.
- **Trauma and surgery:** Prostatectomy, back surgeries,

and spinal cord injuries are among the most common causes.

Since the erection happens in the depth of the erectile tissues, there is no evidence linking the presence of implants or soft tissue fillers in the areolar tissue layer of the penis with organic impotence. However, patients that are overly conscious of their phalloplasty procedure may experience some psychological symptoms, including impotence, especially when they don't fully understand the concept.

Priapism

Contrary to impotence, priapism is a firm, often painful erection that lasts beyond four hours without sexual stimulation. There are two different types of priapism:

Low-flow priapism, the most common, is the result of blood not draining out of the penis. Pain increases progressively as the shaft gets rigid, but the glans remains soft.

High-flow priapism occurs when an excess of blood enters the penis while the drainage remains normal. It is typically painless, and the penis gets erected but not completely rigid.

The underlying cause of priapism often cannot be

determined, but several conditions may play a role: sickle cell anemia, leukemia, and other blood diseases.

Priapism results from altered erection mechanisms, and soft tissue fillers, if injected in the correct layer, do not trigger or influence it.

Ejaculation and urination

Ejaculation is the discharge of semen through the urethra and out of the urinary meatus accompanied by an orgasm (rhythmic pelvic contractions and climax) at the end of sexual intercourse or erogenous stimulation.

Similar to ejaculation, urination is the release of urine from the bladder through the urethra and the urinary meatus.

Since the spongy body is softer than the cavernosum tissues, it is crucial to avoid injecting soft tissue fillers along its pathway to prevent collapsing the urethra and obstructing the flow of semen and urine.

Relaxed penis

The average length of the flaccid penis varies considerably between individuals, and it doesn't correlate to its size during erection. Men who don't shrink much during penile relaxation are known as "showers," while others whose penis grows substantially compared with their relaxed size are known as "growers."

"Showers" have more collagen fibers and more connective tissue, so when the blood drains out their erectile organs, the penis shrinks less than in their counterparts. Injectable fillers composed of microspheres that promote collagen growth will lessen the shrinking of the relaxed penis, turning patients into less retractive "showers."

Scrotum dynamics

The scrotum has two primary functions: protection and temperature control. The testicles need a slightly lower temperature than the body to function correctly. Under cold, stress, or fear, the muscle fibers of the scrotum contract to protect or increase the temperature of the testicles. In situations where the temperature of the testicles gets too warm, the scrotum relaxes to cool them down.

Morphology

Like fingerprints, there are no two identical penises. Of course, some resemblances exist between ethnic groups and family members, but every penis has its specific characteristics. It is a widespread belief that the penis of a black person is more likely to be above average in size and girth and that their skin is typically tighter and thicker. Other races are generally reputed to be below or above the average penis size, their foreskin prone to being redundant, glans pointy or bulky, and so on. Guessing doesn't work all the time, but it is almost effortless to predict if a prospective patient is circumcised or not, big or small, depending on their ethnicity, religion, and body type, amongst other hints.

Penile shape variants are endless, so our classification includes only the most common shapes and sizes.

Length of the penis

The human penis is a cylindrically shaped organ that has infinite variations in both length and circumference. The differences occur not only between individuals but also between one individual himself. The penis grows and shrinks at different intensity levels, and there are myriad internal and external factors that will make it change in appearance. We will not complicate measurements using any "bone pressed" or "stretched" techniques for practical purposes. We will only consider measurements during relaxation and full erection using the circumference of the center of the shaft as a standard.

Shape of the penis

Independently from the length and circumference, the human penis is an organ with multiple shapes, which are described with colloquial names:

Cylindrical

The glans and the body are very similar in circumference size. Cylindrical penises come thick and thin, long and short. A long and narrow cylindrical penis belongs to a subcategory known as "pencil penis." All cylindrical penises are good candidates for girth enhancement, as long as the volume of soft tissue filler used is moderate. Since the glans is as thick as the shaft, multiple implants could dwarf it.

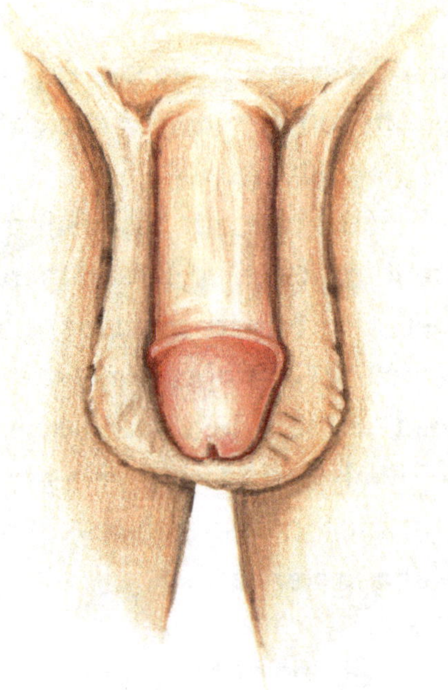

Figure 3.13. Cylindrical penis.

Mushroom

* * *

The mushroom-shaped penis is a variant of the cylindrical penis where the glans is noticeably thicker than the shaft. These patients are the best candidates for girth enhancement since they offer more room for larger implants to increase the width of the shaft without visually dwarfing the size of the glans. Even after significant volume augmentation, these penises often maintain a natural-looking shape.

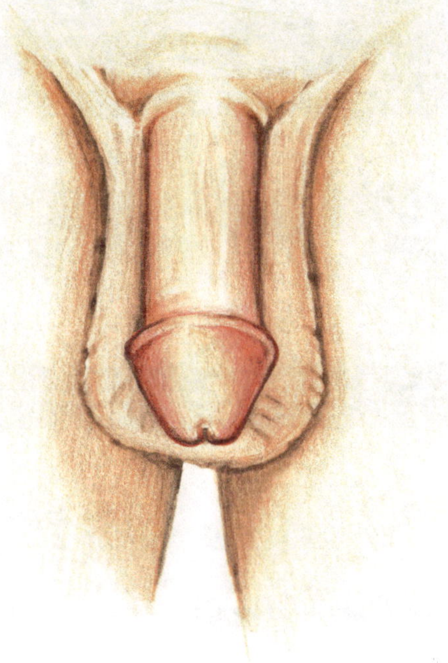

Figure 3.14. Mushroom penis.

Barrel or missile

The penis bulges out in the shaft center while tapering off at both ends. It is a less-than-desirable shape for volume augmentation because the glans will look smaller as the shaft thickens out. In these patients, the correct approach increases the base and leaves the center and the neck untouched, turning the "barrel" into a "truncated cone" shape.

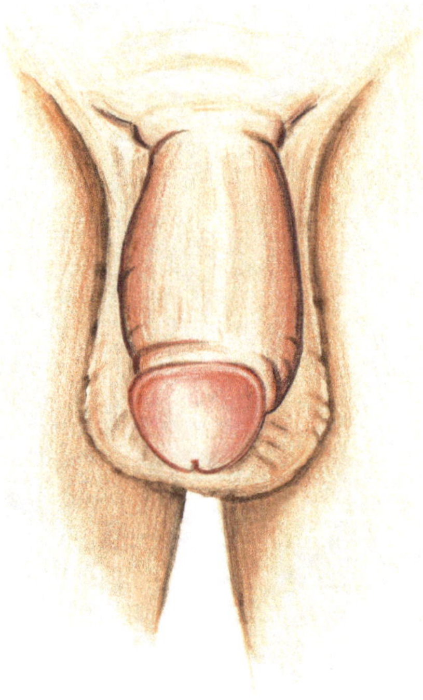

Figure 3.15. Barrel (missile) penis.

Truncated cone or baseball bat

This is a penis that's widest at the neck and tapers back into a thinner base. Widening the bottom and the middle segment of the penis is easy, and the results are often pleasing to the patients.

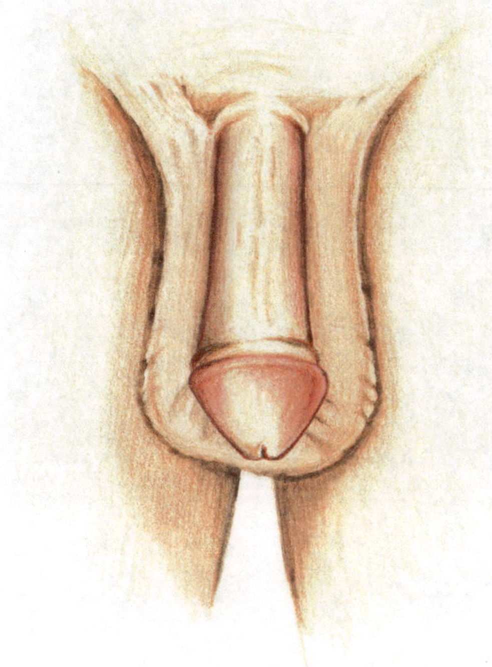

Figure 3.16. Truncated cone penis.

Inverse truncated cone

This is a penis that tapers all the way from a thick base to a medium center to a thin neck. This appearance requires a conservative approach when it comes to girth enhancement, and fillers should only be injected from the middle to the neck of the penis. An overcorrection known as the “pig in a blanket" effect, where the shaft dwarfs the glans, is common in these individuals.

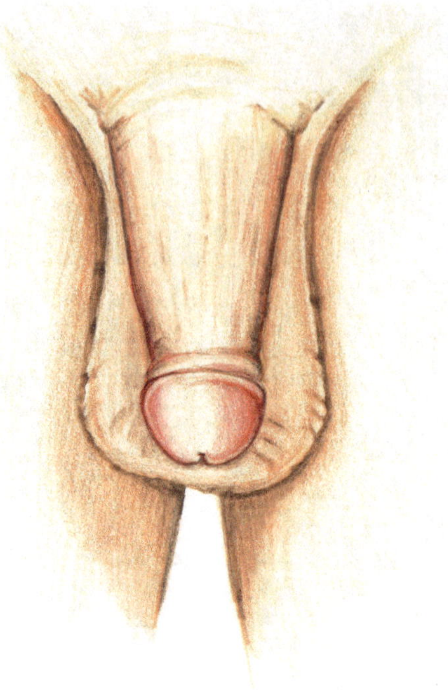

Figure 3.17. Inverse truncated cone penis.

Hourglass

The middle section of this type of penis is slimmer than the top and bottom. It's essentially the inverse of a barrel-shaped penis. The correction of this shape, as well as overall size increases, are easy to do, and the results are pleasing for most patients.

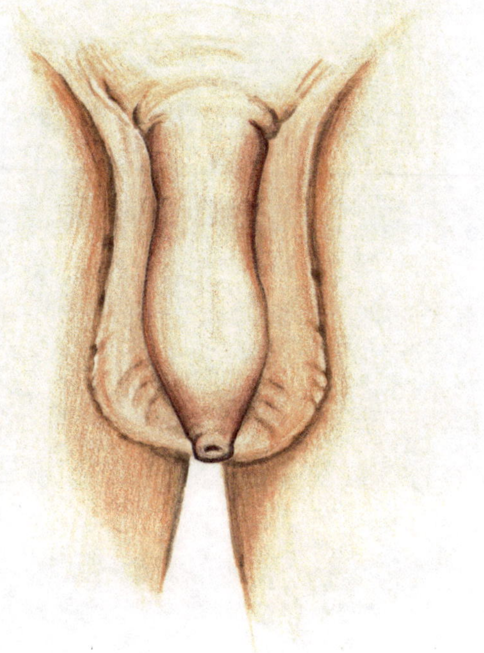

Figure 3.18. Hourglass penis.

Curved

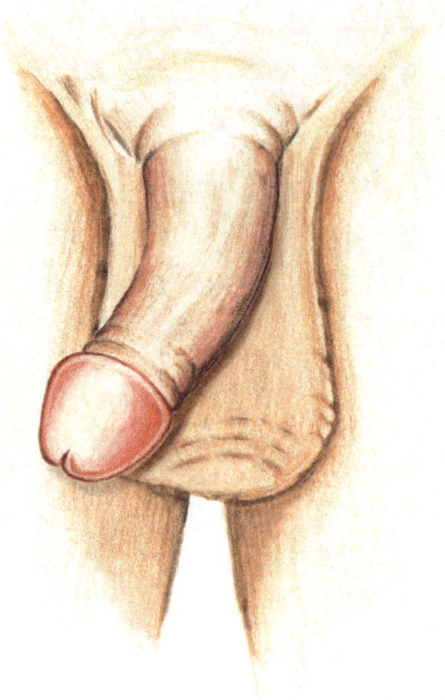

Figure 3.19. Curved penis.

Most penises show some degree of curvature or angulation, which can be upwards, downwards, or to one side, and erection can worsen the condition. Less common variants are S-shaped (multi-curved) and unilateral bulged penises. Light horizontal curvatures can be compensated by adjusting the volume of soft tissue filler (adding more in the concave and less in the convex side), but it should not be attempted if the curvature is intense, an excess of product in one side may create further shape issues. The typical curvature upwards is normal and should not be modified.

* * *

Physical disorders

Micropenis

This term includes both congenital and acquired conditions that result in an abnormally small penis [17]. A micropenis in the adult male is a penis that is 7cm (2¾ inches) or shorter in full erection. The circumference of the shaft is also thin, corresponding with the length.

These patients look for soft tissue fillers as a possible correction, but, unfortunately, the results are disappointing most of the time.

Differentiating a micropenis from a buried penis is essential; see below.

* * *

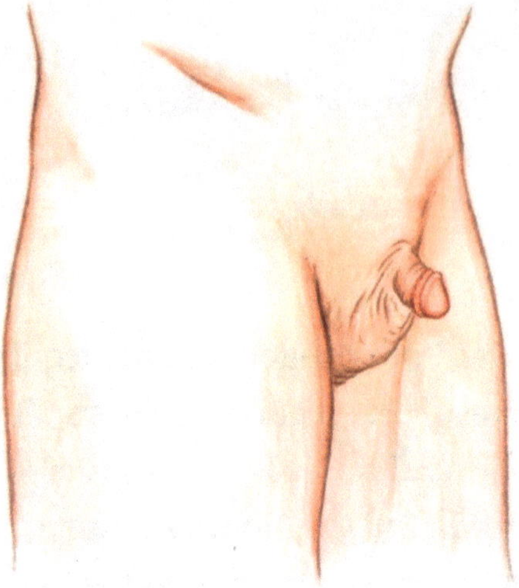

Figure 3.20. Micropenis.

Buried penis

Also known as the hidden penis, a buried penis hides below the surface of the pelvic wall. The penis could actually be average in size, but it is submerged within excess fat tissue, typically in obese patients. Its treatment includes weight control, local liposuction, or reconstructive surgery [18].

* * *

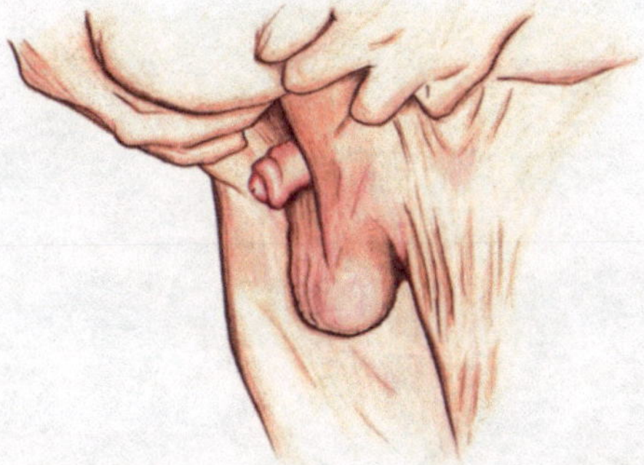

Figure 3.21. Buried penis.

Peyronie's disease

This is a common connective tissue disorder that affects up to 10% of the male population. It is an inflammatory reaction beneath the tunica albuginea which triggers the development of a plaque that causes penile curvature, pain, often erectile dysfunction, loss of girth, and a shortening of the penis. Medical treatments don't seem to be effective, and surgery is usually the best option for this condition [19].

Prospective patients with Peyronie's disease should only be treated with soft tissue fillers if the condition is mild and non-progressive.

* * *

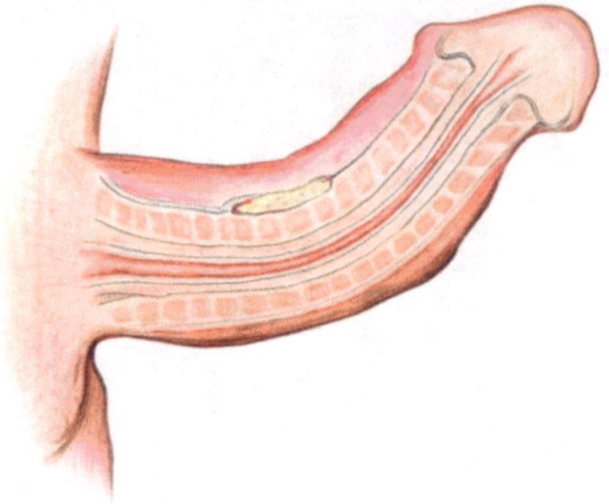

Figure 3.22. Peyronie's disease.

Penoscrotal web

This is a normal condition consisting of an excess of scrotal skin that extends from the front of the scrotum to the mid-to-distal third of the penile shaft. The presence of this redundant skin can create the visual effect of a shorter penis on the undersurface and is a common occurrence in patients who received a low circumcision, which pulls the scrotal skin forward. The surgical removal of this skin flap is a cosmetic procedure that will give the penis a visually more extended appearance without actually modifying the length [20]. The procedure is simple and patients recover quickly, but the area's physical appearance is not always better due to the loss of the otherwise normal skin flap.

* * *

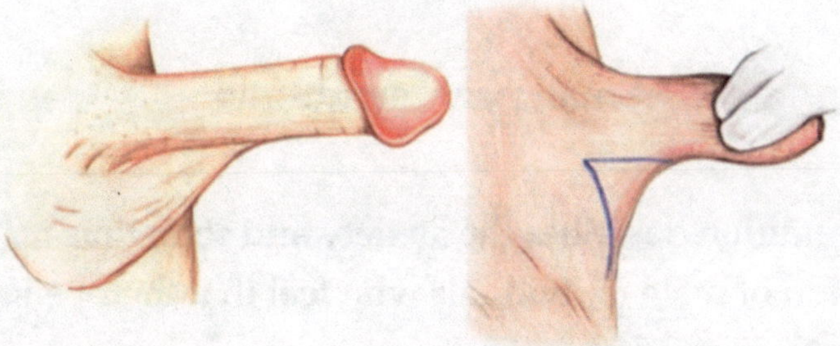

Figure 3.23. Penoscrotal web.

Psychological disorders

Penile dysmorphic disorder

Also known as penile dysmorphophobia, this is a group of psychological and psychiatric conditions where men become so preoccupied with the size or the shape of their penises that it becomes a significant cause of shame or handicap [21]. The following three conditions are examples of penile dysmorphophobia:

The locker room syndrome

Some individuals with this condition are concerned about their penis looking small when observed by other people, even if they don't have an actual size problem. This is typical of guys changing clothes in front of each other, such as in the locker room.

Small penis syndrome

This condition describes the anxiety and sometimes obsession of male individuals who feel that their penis is too small, even when it is average or above average. Patients with the syndrome are different from patients who actually have a below-average sized penis or a condition known as micropenis [22].

Phallocentrism, or phallic identity

This refers to an individual's belief that their penis is the central pillar of their identity. These individuals base their happiness and success in life (amongst other things) on the size and shape of their penis.

The fact is that a large number of male individuals look for options to correct the size or length of their penises, whether they are small or not. In the three conditions mentioned above, patients suffering from "locker room syndrome" and "small penis syndrome" are outstanding candidates for penile girth enhancement, since they see an objective increase in their size and can often easily ignore any resulting imperfections.

In contrast, patients in the third group (phallocentrism)

tend to be picky, are usually unhappy with their results, and are often devastated about minor post-implant flaws.

Remarks

- The penis lacks a coat of subcutaneous fat tissue, otherwise present throughout the body and face. The absence of fat tissue in the penis means that injectable implants are easily visible and palpable. This is independent of the type of soft tissue filler used.

- The penis doesn't have large muscles. The erection comes after the erectile organs get pressure-filled with blood.

- Injectable soft tissue fillers are implanted superficially between the two penile fasciae and away from the erection trigger area around the cavernosum arteries.

- The erectile bodies of the penis (corpora cavernosa and corpus spongiosum) must remain free of soft tissue fillers so their function is not affected. Accidental injections of fillers inside the erectile bodies typically occur when laypersons or inexperienced rough injectors attempt the delicate procedure of penile girth enhancement.

- The glans penis doesn't accept a large volume of soft tissue fillers because its skin is fragile and extremely thin. Underneath that delicate skin lays the spongiosum body, whose cavities connect with the circulatory system. This means injecting soft tissue fillers in this area comes with a high risk of accidental intravascular injections or necrosis by compression.

- Removing the scrotal web gives the penis a visually more extended appearance, but it is only a cosmetic effect that sometimes gives the area an abnormal shape.

- When implanted correctly, soft tissue fillers do not affect the erection mechanisms because there are two layers of tissue between the implant and the erectile bodies: the deep fascia and the tunica albuginea.

- The erection is triggered deep inside the corpora cavernosa and the corpus spongiosum, away from any soft tissue filler implants when they are injected in the correct layer.

- Ejaculation and urination are also not affected with soft tissue fillers, provided that the area where the corpus spongiosum runs remains free of the implant.

- The best candidate for girth enhancement is a circumcised patient with a mushroom-shaped penis.

- The worst candidates for girth enhancement are uncircumcised patients with small, truncated cone or missile-shaped penis and smaller glans, as well as patients with micropenis.

CHAPTER FOUR

Traditional Surgical Techniques

The first attempts at penile elongation and volume augmentation were all surgical, and they all faced different levels of success, as well as complications. At the end of the last century, the arrival of soft tissue fillers brought the new trend of using non-aggressive techniques for penile girth enhancement, offering much better results with less aggressive methods, as the ever-growing demand for these procedures attests.

Some of the surgical techniques discussed in this chapter have become obsolete or are not popular anymore due to their invasive nature and mostly disappointing results. However, I describe them to provide a comparison with the new nonsurgical alternatives.

Fat Injections

This procedure (also known as free fat transfer, or FFT) consists of harvesting fat from the abdomen or another body area through liposuction. The semi-liquid fatty product obtained is then injected into the areolar space of the penis.

Unfortunately, the technique is associated with the death of a large percentage of the fat cells implanted [23], which end up as irregularities, curvatures, asymmetries, nodules, necrosis (death of the implant and / or areas of skin), fatty cysts, calcified fat, granulomas, scars, and insufficient erectile rigidity [24].

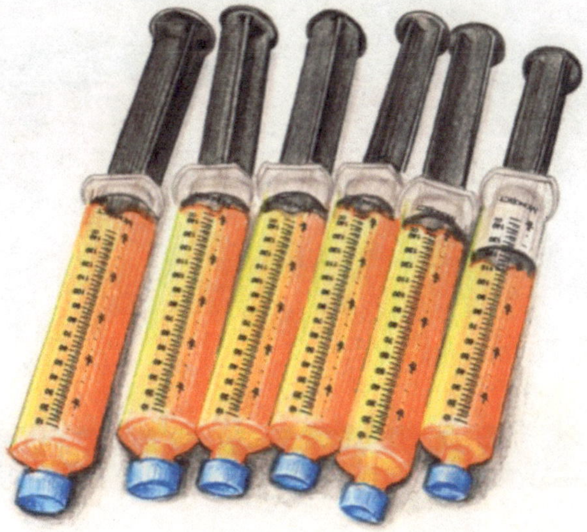

Figure 4.1. Free fat transfer is obtained through liposuction.

Dermal fat grafts

This method consists of transferring blocks of fat tissue cut from one part of the body to a surgically de-gloved (peeled) penis. It is a lengthy procedure with an elevated incidence of complications, such as chronic inflammation of the penis, necrosis, scarring, retraction, and more [25]. The donor site is also not immune to complications, such as the risk of infection and extensive, visible scars.

The penile dermal graft is almost obsolete due to its inconsistent results and a significant rate of complications.

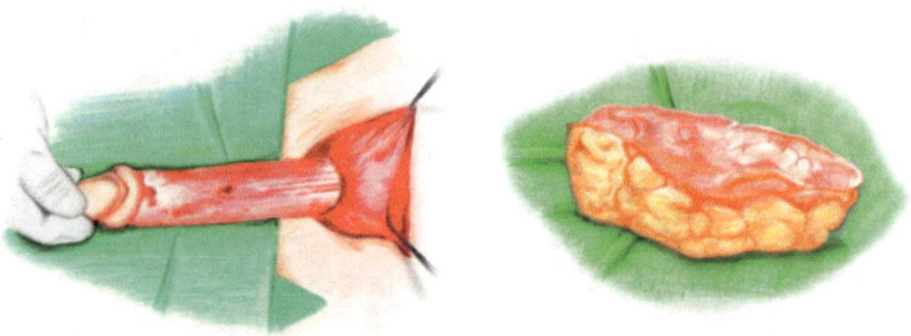

Figure 4.2. Dermal fat graft.

Allografts

Allografts are another procedure that has mostly fallen into disuse. It consists of implanting sheets of donated human skin tissue (Alloderm™) under the skin on a previously surgically de-gloved penis. This scaffolding could provide a more consistent cosmetic result concerning penile symmetry and durability, as well as a lower incidence of adverse effects than with dermal fat grafts [26]. Another advantage that allografts have over dermal fat grafts is that there is no need for a donor-site as well as the fact that the grafts themselves supposedly have a better chance of survival. However, its viability beneath the overlying thin penile skin can be compromised, creating erosion, fibrosis, infection, resorption, and skin loss, affecting penile length and function.

Allografts have their place, and they work well for other indications, but they are not an adequate solution for penile girth enhancement. Even its manufacturer warns against its use in penile augmentation.

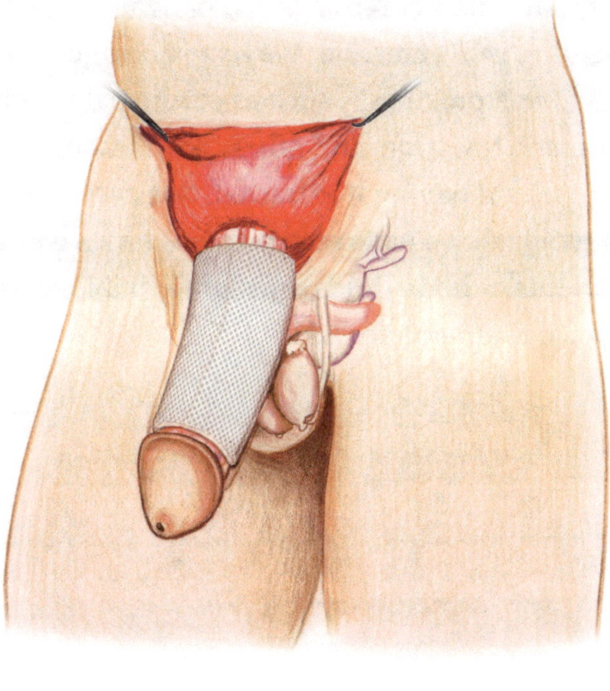

Figure 4.3. Allograft.

Subcutaneous soft silicone implants

A product inspired by penile scaffoldings is a soft, medical-grade silicone prosthesis implanted surgically under the skin of the penis through an incision in the pubic area. Before re-stitching the skin, the prosthesis is affixed to the pubic tissues and the neck of the penis. This procedure has been reported as safe and efficient by isolated authors [27], but it is possibly the most controversial penile enhancement surgical technique offered at the moment.

These implants are not retractile, so patients end up with a permanently visible erection. We have documented several reactions to this prosthesis, such as severe pain, protrusion of the implant, infection, and other complications which led to the patient having it extracted. But even after surgical removal, we have seen seromas (cysts containing large amounts of body fluids), unsightly pubic scars, retraction, and other deformities.

* * *

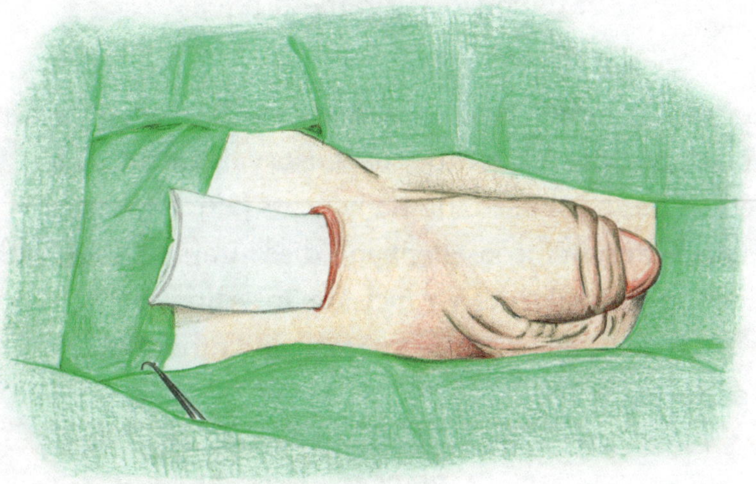

Figure 4.4. Soft silicone implant.

Other penile enhancement techniques

Austoni [28] described a method consisting of a bilateral venous graft transplantation to augment the cavernous bodies of the penis in an attempt to correct deformities associated with Peyronie's disease. This technique also increases penile girth size during the erect state but is not standard for girth enhancement.

Surgical penile elongation

The only effective techniques for penile elongation are surgical, so we will mention these basic concepts before moving on to discuss the nonsurgical procedures.

Suspensory ligament release

The most common types of surgical penile elongation are procedures that release the suspensory ligament. This method has been used for many years [29], however, results are often inconsistent and discouraging, even with advancements like the VY incision, insertions of vascularized flaps, silicone spacers, and other tissue expanders.

A new product called MEDPOR, made of high-density, porous polyethylene seems to be a good alternative for elongation when inserted between the internal end of the cavernous bodies and the pubis. It supposedly results in a one-third increase in penile length [30]. However, there is not much of a sample size of this procedure at the moment, but if the gains are even half of what they claim it would be an excellent alternative to the classical approach.

Penile elongation surgeries often leave visible scars that can be large and deforming, and satisfaction rates tend to be low. So there is a need to explore other methods and directions to achieve therapeutic success.

In simple terms, the release of the suspensory ligament offers three possible results that make it questionable [31]:

- Moderate gains.
- No gains.

• Retraction and shortening.

Pubic liposuction & panniculectomy

These extra-genital surgical procedures offer a visually longer penis without actually altering its physical size.

As we previously mentioned, overweight individuals develop a thick fat pad in the pubic area, creating a condition known as the buried or hidden penis. Patients may not be able to carry out regular hygiene, direct the urine stream, or be sexually active due to the condition.

Although these patients are obese, weight loss often does not fully reverse the problem, as the fat pad may remain unchanged.

The most common procedure for correcting the buried penis is the liposuction of the pubic fat pad. Still, patients with extreme conditions may require supra-pubic lipectomy or panniculectomy [32].

Ventral phalloplasty

This is a simple surgical procedure designed to correct the penoscrotal web, a typical condition consisting of an excess of scrotal skin that extends from the scrotum to the mid-to-distal third of the penile shaft. The presence of this redundant skin can create the visual effect of a shorter penis on its undersurface, and it is a common occurrence in patients who received a distal (low) circumcision which pulls the penile skin forward. The surgical removal of this skin flap is a simple cosmetic procedure that will give the penis a visually extended appearance [33].

Glans enhancement

Surgical glans enhancement with scaffoldings has never been a very successful procedure, and nonsurgical soft tissue fillers also lack promise. Attempts at enhancing the glans with different soft tissue fillers, like Hyaluronic Acid [34], cross-linked dextran spheres [35], silicone micro-droplets, and others have proven successful to some extent. However, the approach must be conservative to prevent accidental intravascular injections or local necrosis and scaring, which are frequent complications.

Glans enhancement is questionable whether the soft tissue filler is deposited strictly into the thin skin covering the glans or injected into the depth of the spongy body that lays directly under it. Inserting any soft tissue filler into the spongy body produces rapid migration through the venous system, and thrombosis, necrosis, scarring, retraction, and deformity are common complications.

Scrotal enhancement

Scrotal enlargement can be surgical, with the insertion of

testicular prosthesis, or non-surgical, with soft tissue fillers. Injectable substances to enlarge the scrotum go back to the early ninety-forties using different materials, such as silicone oil and saline solution. However, the surgical alternative (implants of silicone prosthesis) continues to be a popular and well-tolerated procedure [36].

Tolerance and longevity seem good for both alternatives, with the most common side effects being retraction of the scrotum in some individuals and nodulation of the soft tissue filler.

Scrotal Relaxation is a temporary nonsurgical solution for the overly retracting scrotum. Known as "scrotox," it consists of botulinum toxin injections that relax both the cremaster and the dartos muscles, creating a drop of the testicular bag and the testicles.

Foreskin restoration

It is an uncommon, almost fictional procedure that delivers unpleasant and discouraging results most of the time (if not always). The natural foreskin is a flap of very elastic skin to accommodate the penis during erection and cover the glans in the relaxed state. Unfortunately, even though there are new and old reports of success with this practice [37], there is no ideal method for restoring it — not even taking a graft from an acceptable donor site in the body. The healing process also creates scars that interfere with the area and the whole penis's normal function.

CHAPTER FIVE
Soft Tissue Fillers

Nonsurgical male enhancement procedures mainly refer to injectable soft tissue fillers to augment the volume of the penile shaft, the glans, or the scrotum.

Compared to surgical procedures, injectable soft tissue fillers have dramatically diminished the frequency and severity of complications associated with surgery. The modern approach is much safer, spearheading a new trend towards non-invasive, in-office procedures that avoid hospitalization, general anesthesia, incisions, drains, stitches, prolonged downtime, and permanent scars.

Soft tissue fillers are substances used to create a fuller appearance in the body area where they're injected. They have been used for decades for the face, but new indications include other body areas, such as the hands, penis, and scrotum.

Choosing the correct soft tissue filler for the different male enhancement procedures is probably the most critical decision for both the physician and the patient. Both parties must understand the science behind them, and prospective patients should know their essential characteristics before authorizing their use inside their bodies.

The safety and efficacy of a soft tissue filler depends on three main factors that are intertwined to give the final results:

- The injection technique.
- The physical and chemical characteristics of the product.
- The response of the host's tissues.

These three factors must be favorable for the result to be safe and effective; if one of them fails, the implant is unsatisfactory or complicated.

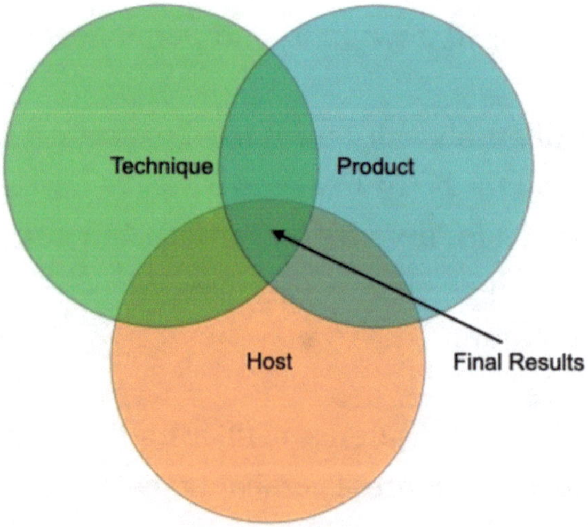

Figure 5.1. Interacting factors for safety and efficacy of a soft

tissue filler implant.

To start, let's look at some examples: years ago, when soft tissue fillers became popular, a known patient requested injections of a specific product for her wrinkles. Knowing that she was a strict vegetarian, I explained that the brand of her choice contained bovine collagen, and she couldn't believe that her request involved injections of something she wouldn't even eat.

Another patient was interested in a heavily advertised, home-brewed product developed for penile enhancement by a layperson. When I did a cursory internet search, I discovered that its name was better known as an electric bike brand and I found no registered soft tissue filler under that name. Further research revealed that it was an illegal silicone product used by impostors.

Choosing the most appropriate soft tissue filler should not be taken lightly. It is crucial to know their composition, time of effect, interaction with the surrounding tissues and the body in general. Also, it should be manufactured by a well-known, ethical manufacturer.

Other important facts to consider are the possible consequences of their use, especially long-term, and the best corrective options if something goes wrong.

This chapter focuses on the benefits and pitfalls of the most popular soft tissue fillers, trying to help prospective patients reach their best decisions. The list of authorized soft tissue fillers is long and keeps growing, and it is necessary to classify them so we can have a better understanding of what they are and how they work.

Let's start with the two main groups: one based on the permanency of the fillers in the tissues (longevity) and the other based on the primary substance's physical characteristics.

Longevity

There are three groups of products based on the amount of time that they remain in human tissues:

- Temporary or absorbable (around one year).
- Long-lasting or slowly absorbable (one to four years).
- Permanent or non-absorbable.

Physical characteristics

This is important because products differ significantly from each other, and their physical characteristics are critical to their mechanism of action, final results, and possible side effects:

- Fast absorbable gel.

- Slowly absorbable microspheres.
- Non-absorbable microspheres.

Gel-based soft tissue fillers

Gels, such as hyaluronic acid (HA), were introduced at the end of the last century and are the most common soft tissue fillers. Most of them are made of hyaluronic acid and are available under many different brand names. Unlike microsphere-based products that promote collagen, gels remain in the tissues in their original form and create augmentation by holding water, which expands the neighboring tissues [38]. The body does not develop any new vascular tissue inside hyaluronic acid gel implants and no blood or body defenses can enter into their core, making them prone to infection.

One good attribute of hyaluronic acid is that it can be dissolved with injections of the enzyme hyaluronidase, a quick solution for patients that are not happy with their results.

Among the long list of available hyaluronic acid-based products comes Voluma® and Volux® (Allergan), the favorites for penile girth enhancement due to their viscosity and longevity.

Hyaluronic acid is absorbed in months, and patients need touch-up sessions for as long as they want to keep the effects.

If used in large volumes, gels can give the penis a "spongy" feel for some time, and imperfections, such as shifting, bumps, and voids are common in this group.

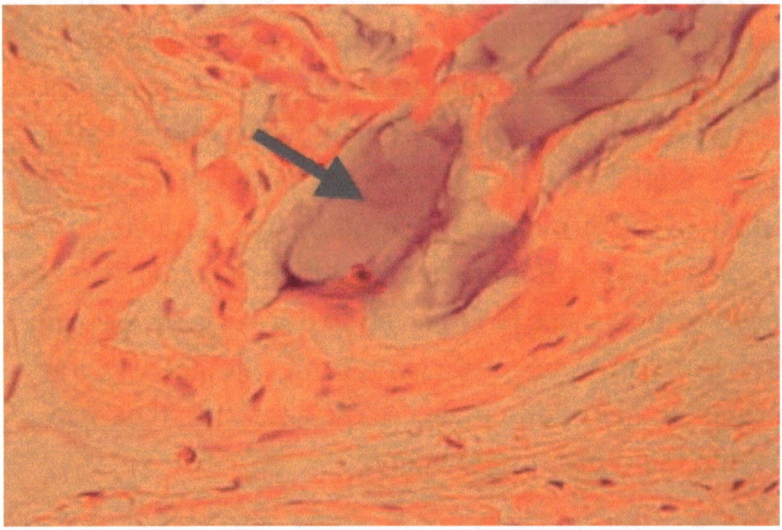

Figure 5.2. Micrograph showing hyaluronic acid gel in human tissues.

Solid microsphere-based soft tissue fillers

These products contain solid microspheres suspended in a gelatinous vehicle. After the injection, the vehicle (or carrier) is absorbed and the microspheres remain in the tissues, triggering the formation of the patient's collagen around them, ultimately increasing the area's volume. Think about sand grains turning into pearls inside of an oyster.

These implants have the advantage of promoting collagen growth and new tiny arteries and veins around them, creating what some authors call "living implants" [39, 40], which integrate nicely into the area and behave like native tissue [41,42].

There are two main groups of microspheres:

1) Slowly absorbable or biodegradable:
• Calcium hydroxyapatite (Radiesse®, Merz Aesthetics);
• Polycaprolactone (Ellansé®, Sinclair Pharma).

2) Permanent or non-biodegradable:
• Polymethylmethacrylate, or PMMA (Linnea Safe® and Linnea Avanti®, Laboratorio Lebon; Bellafill®, Suneva).

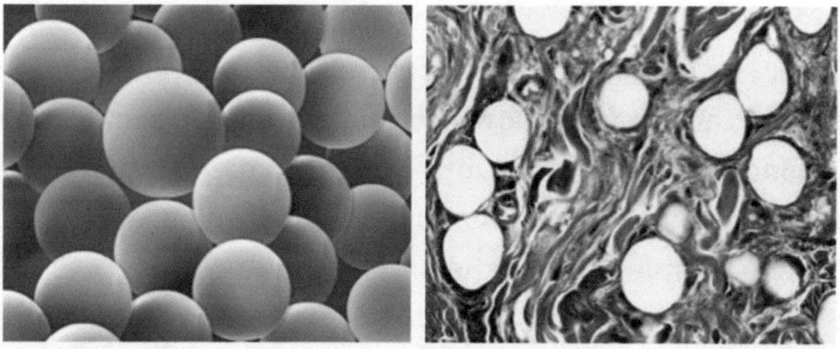

Figure 5.3. Micrograph showing PMMA microspheres in human tissues.

Combined products

* * *

Bellafill® is manufactured in San Diego, CA, and is approved by the US FDA. It is an excellent choice for facial procedures, but, unfortunately, the bovine collagen in this product makes it less than desirable for the specific demands of phalloplasty. Bellafill® contains a ratio of 20% PMMA microspheres and 80% bovine collagen, and, due to the bovine collagen, this product requires an allergy skin test before its use.

After Bellafill is injected, the collagen remains like a gel for months, and the solid PMMA microspheres remain in the tissues permanently. It has been proven safe and efficacious for most facial areas, like the nose, cheeks, and jawline. Even though it has been approved by the US FDA since 2006, it's still the new kid in the block for penile girth enhancement, and clinical trials need to be conducted to prove its safety and efficacy.

Other combinations of two or more substances are less popular, and little is known about their use for penile girth enhancement. Therefore, my strong recommendation is to avoid them until there is enough research and a large enough sample size of patients.

The medical community prefers single fillers made of only one active product, as they are more predictable and have fewer potential side effects coming from their interaction.

Oil-based soft tissue fillers

This section is discussed as a warning, not as a recommendation.

The use of liquid injectable silicone oil for cosmetic purposes dates back to the nineteen-forties. Still, it has always raised controversial opinions regarding its efficacy and serious concerns about its long-term safety.

The large volume needed to achieve a noticeable increase in penile size comes with a list of immediate and, most pertinently, long-term known complications: rejection, migration, chronic granuloma, discoloration, hardening of the skin, ulceration, and more [43].

Migration of oil-based soft tissue fillers can happen over months and years, and gravity creates a movement of the oil to the distal sections of the penis, abnormally thickening the foreskin or making a bell-shaped penis in circumcised patients.

Low-volume silicone injections gained popularity when Jones and other authors published their experience using small amounts of the product and a micro-droplet injection technique to treat HIV-associated facial atrophy [44].

Yacobi et al. [45] reported serial injections of smaller amounts of silicone to increase the penile circumference by an average of 2.6 cm (around 1 inch) in 324 patients. However, their results seem too optimistic since they reported that all patients were fully satisfied without any reported short-term complications. Some of them even reported better erections and control of their premature ejaculation. The main problem with this study is that the follow-up time was only 36 months, and it is known that silicone complications tend to happen many years later. Hopefully, those patients can maintain the same level of satisfaction and lack of side effects years after the injections.

To put it succinctly, the use of silicone oil with the micro-droplet technique for girth and glans enhancement has not been explored sufficiently. It seems to be that the safest area for its use is the face, contrary to the penis, which has shown a higher level of complications.

Silicone oil is also the great impostor of phalloplasty. It is common to find false advertising and claims using names that give the impression of being one of the ethical products mentioned earlier in this chapter. Titles like "super-collagen," "hyaluronic acid with growth factors," private brands of "PMMA," and others are designed to trick uneducated or naive patients.

Except for temporary authorization for HIV-associated lipoatrophy treatment almost two decades ago [46], silicone oil hasn't been approved as a soft tissue filler.

* * *

We strongly discourage prospective patients from using silicone oil for nonsurgical phalloplasty or any other indication.

Soft tissue fillers used for phalloplasty

To simplify my information and the plethora of choices, I will only discuss the three most popular products for phalloplasty based on medical facts and doctor / patient preferences.

Hyaluronic Acid (HA)

HA is the most popular soft tissue filler in aesthetic medicine, and there are a wide variety of concentrations, presentations, and brands. It is safe, reversible, and suitable for facial treatments but not the best choice for phalloplasty. However, it is the most popular product at the moment because it is available worldwide.

- Physical characteristics: Gel.
- Longevity: Short-lasting.
- Brand: Voluma® (Allergan) and many others.
- Pros: Very well tolerated, reversible.
- Cons: Short-lived, prone to shifting, gives the penis a soft and spongy feel.

Polycaprolactone (PCL)

This is the newest product of the three discussed here. It has the advantage of being a microsphere-based product that produces a firm, natural-feeling implant. In addition to that, it is slowly absorbable, which gives peace of mind to patients that are not comfortable with permanent bodily modifications. Along with permanent PMMA, polycaprolactone — in products such as Ellansé® — is one of the two most popular choices for phalloplasty where it is available.

• Physical characteristics: Microspheres.
• Longevity: Long-lasting (one to four years, depending on the variety used).
• Brand: Ellansé® ; it comes in three versions based on longevity: L (3 years), M (2 years), S (1 year). Version E (4 years) is available in Europe.
• Pros: Natural feel, long-lasting effects.
• Cons: Nodules, voids, or other irregularities that disappear as the carrier absorbs.

Polymethylmethacrylate (PMMA)

This is the oldest of the three products and the choice for patients looking for permanent results. As a microsphere-based product, it produces a firm, natural-feeling implant that lasts for life.

• Physical characteristics: Microspheres.
• Longevity: Permanent.
• Brand: Linnea Safe® and Linnea Avanti®.

• Pros: Natural feel, creates a permanent "living implant."
• Cons: Prone to create voids and nodules; removal by surgical extraction only.

	Chemical Name	Physical Characteristics	Brands
Non absorbable	Polymethylmethacrylate PMMA	Microspheres	Linnea Safe® Linnea Avanti®
Slowly absorbable	Calcium hydroxylapatite CaHA		Radiesse®
	Polycaprolactone PCL		Ellansé®
	Dextran		Lippen® D
Absorbable	Hyaluronic acid HA	Gel	Voluma® and multiple brands
Combinations	PMMA + Bovine collagen	Microspheres + Gel	Bellafil®

Table 5.1. Most popular soft tissue fillers used for phalloplasty.

Ethical use of soft tissue fillers

Silicone oil is possibly the best-known impostor, often offered with names that imply collagen, hyaluronic acid, or PMMA. Be suspicious if you see any of the following conditions on the label or in the appearance of a soft tissue filler:

• Not a familiar brand or a "private brand" that doesn't appear on internet searches.

• Bulky products: home-brewed silicone oil comes in half or one-liter size bottles.
• Product labels with extraordinary statements, such as "super collagen," "PMMA with growth factors," etc. Health authorities do not authorize legends that claim superlative and extreme results.
• Unprofessional, homemade packaging.
• Lack of an adhesive label with the basic information of the product.

The following guidelines must be observed by ethical physicians using soft tissue fillers:

1) Hand out the product to the patient for close inspection.
2) The product must be in its original, sealed packaging.
3) Syringes are taken out of their sealed package in front of the patient.
4) Each syringe or kit has an adhesive label with the product information; it must be kept in the patient's file and, ideally, a second label should be given to the patient for his personal records.
5) The label indicates the brand, lot number, expiration date, and the manufacturer's name and contact information. The label should be original, sometimes with a barcode or hologram.

It is important to have the product's information as a reference for future needs, such as if a consultation with another physician or practice is needed down the road.

CHAPTER SIX

Selection of candidates

Male enhancement procedures are now popular and highly desirable, but they are not for everybody. There are ideal candidates and suitable candidates, but there is also a large number of prospects that, for different reasons, will not qualify for genitalia modification.

The ideal candidate

The perfect patient for girth enhancement meets most of the following criteria:

- Good health
- Age between 25 and 60 years old.
- Circumcised.
- Penis longer than 7.5 cm (3") during full erection.
- Lean pubic fat pad.
- Non-retractive penis.
- Psychologically sound and stable.
- Realistic goals (increase of 1.2–2.5 cm or 0.5 – 1").
- Financially solvent.

Prospective patients who don't fulfill the entire list can still be accepted, provided they do not fall into any categories that make them non-acceptable.

The conditional candidate

The following conditions may require a medical evaluation before deciding if the patient is the right for a girth enhancement procedure:

- Uncircumcised.
- Peyronie's disease.
- Congenital or acquired malformations, including micropenis.
- Extreme obesity.
- Buried penis.
- Penile prosthesis, hard or soft silicone subcutaneous implants (scaffoldings).
- Inflatable pumps.
- History of trauma, surgery, scars, active lesions.
- Previous use of soft tissue fillers.
- Chronic, degenerative, autoimmune, or metabolic diseases; especially if they are not well controlled.
- Co-existing conditions like diabetes, cirrhosis, chemotherapy, HIV infection.
- Smoking, alcoholism, use or abuse of recreational drugs.
- Disapproval of his sexual partner.
- Religious implications.
- Financial hardship.

Prospective patients that are not accepted

Many conditions disqualify potential phalloplasty patients.

The most common ones are listed below:

- Prior treatments with silicone oil injections or unknown substances.
- Multi-treated individuals with scars, tissue damage, deformity.
- Phallocentrism: unrealistic expectations, looking for extreme results, obsessive behavior towards the penis.
- Dismorphophobia: individuals that won't tolerate irregularities or are obsessively worried about future complications.

Other considerations for patient screening

Although not a universal idea, some medical practices suggest that uncircumcised prospects have a distal (low) and tight circumcision — with the surgical scar near the neck and head of the penis — three months before their nonsurgical phalloplasty procedure.

Prospects under medical supervision or treatment must have the approval of their treating physician before undergoing nonsurgical phalloplasty treatment.

Measuring the penis

There are many systems and techniques to measure the penis, and they have appeared in multiple studies, clinical trials, scientific websites, forums, and books. However, it is a simple yet complicated task due to the penile size variations in response to a substantial number of stimuli.

It is essential to record the basal measurements of the penis to assess the girth enhancement treatment progress and understand the potential limitations. The medical office will record your measurements every time to assess and track the evolution of the treatment.

Relaxed Penis

Place the ruler on top of the penis before any signs of arousal and without manipulating it. While maintaining the ruler in its place, hold out the penis and record the size. After that, manually stretch to its maximum length and log the result again. Then take a measurement of the circumference, typically at the center of the shaft.

Recording both relaxed and extended measurements provides an idea of how retractile the penis is, which helps decide the specific post-care treatment.

Erected penis

During a full erection place the rigid ruler on top of the penis and gently press the pubic fat pad to obtain the length. Then get the circumference of the penis by placing the measuring tape around the thickest area, typically mid-shaft. Longer penises require girth measurements at the base, center, and neck.

Repeat the measuring process at least two times per day for several days and record the average numbers.

Uncircumcised versus circumcised

The ideal candidate for girth enhancement is a circumcised patient. Two tight membranes (the tunica albuginea and Buck's deep fascia) englobe the erectile structures of the penis. On top of them lies a 'bag' of skin that is firm in circumcised but very loose in uncircumcised individuals.

Implanting any filler into the loose "bag" at the areolar space level in an uncircumcised patient is challenging. Migration, shifting, and product clumping are common, and there is a high risk of soft tissue migration or accidental injection into the foreskin that can interfere with the aesthetics and dynamics of the area and the penis as a whole.

Uncircumcised patients seeking more substantial increases are encouraged to have a distal (low) and tight circumcision performed three months before their girth enhancement procedure. Uncircumcised patients that have received soft tissue fillers can get circumcised as long as the implant has settled and that the soft tissue filler is positively identified.

Psychological aspects

Men who undergo penile augmentation for various mental and sexual reasons appear to be satisfied with the results. They often experience improved attitudes and reduce the psychological distress surrounding the penis. In general, they also seem to experience an increase in their overall self-esteem [47].

For most men, their penis size reflects their masculinity, and a real or imaginary small penis can associate with depression, anxiety, low body image, impaired quality of life, erectile dysfunction, and other psychological issues [48].

On the other side of the psychological spectrum is the ideal super male, with an above-average penis size, athletic figure, and a handsome face. But even with all these attributes, some still depend on their penis size to be happy, socially accepted, and prosperous. As a result, they are probably the worst candidates for penile girth enhancement because the outcome of a procedure can be devastating if it doesn't meet their expectations.

Lever [13] reported that men with a larger-than-average penis are more satisfied with their appearance, suggesting a possible confidence effect of perceived large penis size.

Small penis syndrome

* * *

One of the most significant psychological issues regarding penis size is the "small penis syndrome," which is when patients with an average or even big penis become obsessed with compulsive checking rituals, body dysmorphic disorder, and excessive concern over having a "small" penis. These patients are among the best candidates for penile girth enhancement with soft tissue fillers because they can immediately see a more massive penis. Often, their gains opaque their imperfections because they tend to focus on volume more than on aesthetics.

Previous surgeries and pre-existing malformations

Some patients will not stop in their desire to have a bigger penis. They will request more sessions than usual and won't listen to the advice to stay on the conservative side. Other patients that have had procedures already will find a new technique or a new product and want to jump on it, ignoring the scars, retractions, even accidents that they've gone through with other methods.

Patients with previous male enhancement procedures or with scars and deformities left by surgery, manipulation, and accidents must openly disclose and discuss these with the doctor as far in advance as possible. It is common to see that these patients won't take "no" as an option.

Peyronie's Disease

* * *

This is a disorder of the connective tissue resulting from the growth of fibrous plaques and scarring forming in the tunica albuginea that causes abnormal curvature, erectile dysfunction, localized loss of girth, and pain in the penis.

Its course is not entirely predictable [49] and it's not known if injecting soft tissue fillers at such a level will affect the disease's progression. For that reason, patients must discuss their plans with their urologist or the professional controlling the condition before attempting any elective cosmetic procedure on their penis. Even if the patients get their authorization, they should consider that there are no clinical trials that prove the safety of soft tissue fillers when their Peyronie's disease is in progress.

Since there is not enough information, our best recommendation is that patients with active Peyronie's disease should not get any soft tissue filler injections unless the condition is mild and non-progressive.

Previous penile implants

Alloderm®, soft silicone scaffoldings, solid silicone implants, inflatable pumps placed inside the corpora cavernosa, and a history of other surgical treatments require a live assessment before deciding if it’s safe to add soft tissue fillers.

Realistic expectations

The ratios of length vs. girth and penile shaft vs. glans of the penis must be considered to maintain its natural appearance after the implant of soft tissue fillers.

As mentioned before in this book, the best candidates to receive a higher volume of soft tissue fillers are patients with a "mushroom" shaped penis, where the glans is substantially more prominent than the circumference of the shaft.

Amongst the less desirable candidates are patients with a "missile" shaped penis, where both the shaft and the glans taper down from the middle section of the penis. In these patients, even small amounts of filler will distort the appearance by dwarfing the glans.

Most patients with an average-sized penis should not expect more than 1.25 cm (0.5") if they want to preserve their normal appearance. However, in real life, the majority wants to achieve gains of 2.5 cm (1”) or more.

The patient also needs to realize that penile implants are currently far from perfect. Realistically, patients should expect a reasonable number of imperfections, such as voids or small nodules, which can be corrected to some extent through further touch-up sessions or spontaneously if the filler is absorbable.

Age restrictions

Penile girth enhancement is an elective procedure that can be temporary or permanent, depending on the soft tissue filler used. In theory, patients of legal adult age can have this procedure. Still, it is recommended to use absorbable fillers in young adults since their lifestyle and ideas could change dramatically. Permanent fillers seem to be a good option for patients older than 25 who are well informed about the procedure and the soft tissue filler being used. Patients interested in girth enhancement with permanent soft tissue fillers should also always have the approval of their sexual partners.

Preliminary self-assessment

Since there are benefits, known complications, and pitfalls associated with male enhancement techniques, it is necessary to assess the candidate from all possible angles, including anatomical, physiological, and psychological conditions.

A preliminary self-assessment is helpful to give prospective patients a good idea of the main topics that they must discuss at the time of their initial consultation with their physician.

The following table summarizes the inclusion/exclusion criteria mentioned at the beginning of this chapter.

Ideal	Less than ideal
Good health	Uncircumcised
Age 25 - 60	Peyrone's disease or other conditions
Circumcised	Congenital or acquired malformations
Penis longer than 7.5 cm (3") in full erection	Micropenis
Lean pubic fat pad	History of penile prosthesis or scaffoldings
Non-retractive penis	History of inflatable pumps
Psychologically stable	Surgeries, scars, active lesions
Realistic goals	History of use of known soft tissue fillers
Informed sexual partner	Coexisting chronic diseases
	Financial hardship

Patients who do not qualify
Previous use of injectable silicone oil or other unknown substances
Multi-treated individuals: surgeries, implants, accidents, deformities, etc.
Phallocentrism: unrealistic and exaggerated expectations; obsessive behavior towards the penis
Dismorphophobia: Intolerance to irregularities or obsessive preoccupation for possible future complications

Table 6.1. Patient selection criteria.

CHAPTER SEVEN
Nonsurgical phalloplasty techniques

Since medicine can be more of an art than an exact science, physicians use a wide diversity of methods and techniques in phalloplasty, often created or modified to suit their personal needs. This chapter discusses the most common approach used by the author.

Drawing the work plan

One way to achieve a smooth and homogeneous implant is by dividing the penis into sections and marking the area with a surgical pen [7,50].

First, two longitudinal lines are drawn on the ventral side to delimit the path of the corpus spongiosum. This area must be free of soft tissue filler to avoid interference with urination or ejaculation (Figure 7.1).

Then two other longitudinal lines are drawn at 2 and 10 o'clock (Figure 7.2). After that, two or three equidistant transverse lines are drawn to divide the dorsal and lateral surfaces of the penis into 6, 9, or 12 segments, according to the organ's length (Figure 7.3).

Subsequently, two or three entry points are opened per

side so that the cannula freely reaches each segment. This can be done with the help of an injection gun (Figure 7.4) or manually using the original syringe of the soft tissue filler (Figure 7.5).

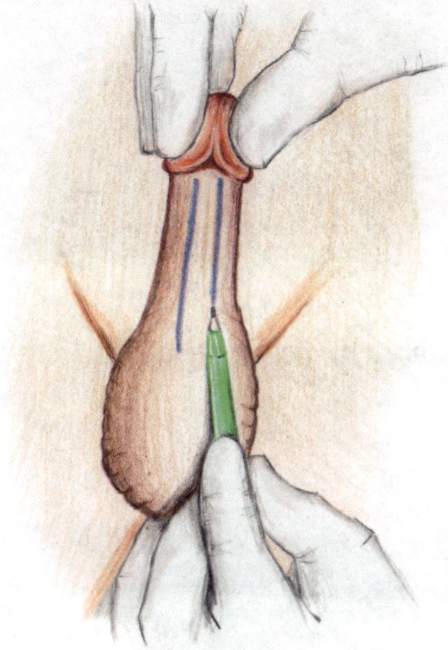

Figure 7.1. Delimiting the corpus spongiosum.

* * *

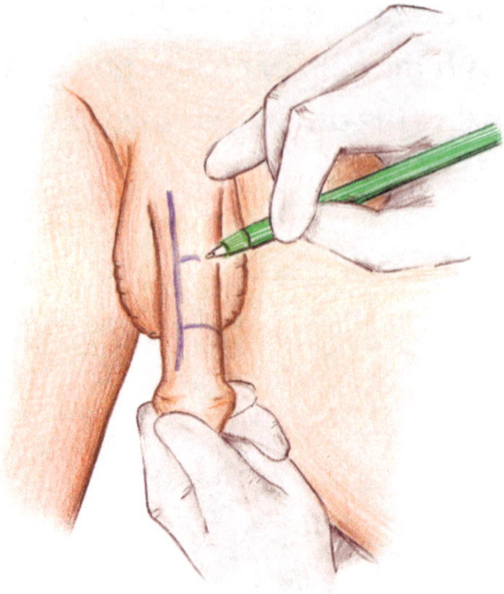

Figure 7.2. Drawing the dorsal segments.

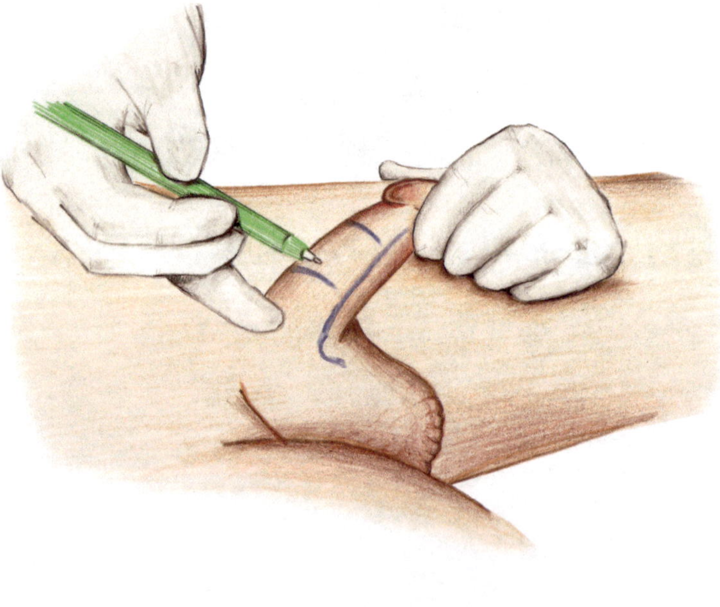

Figure 7.3. Drawing the lateral segments.

* * *

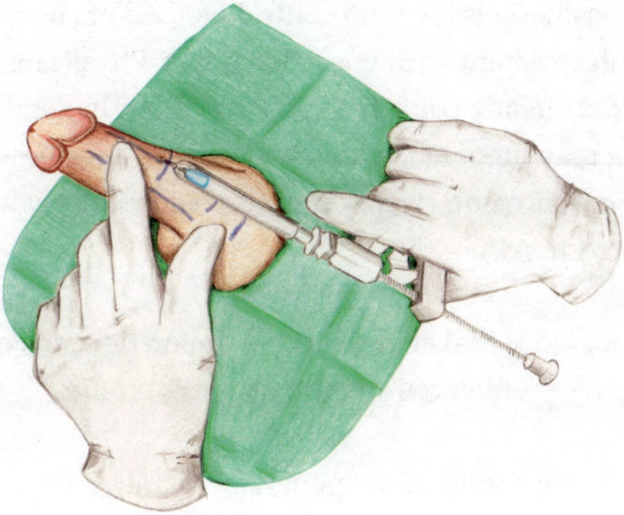

Figure 7.4. Implanting the soft tissue filler with an injection gun.

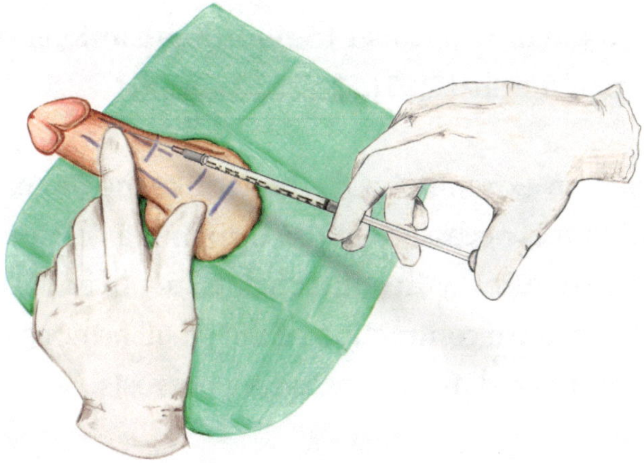

Figure 7.5. Implanting the soft tissue filler through manual injections.

Anesthesia

* * *

Local anesthesia is the pain control method of choice for girth enhancement with injectable fillers. Physicians using fillers that already contain a local anesthetic in their formula may prepare the area with topical anesthesia (cream or ointment) twenty minutes before the beginning of the injections.

Supplementary oral analgesia or sedation depends on the physician's preferences and the patient's profile.

The sensitive nerves of the penis run mainly on top of the cavernous bodies between the tunica albuginea and the deep fascia (Figure 2.3). First, the two dorsal nerves are blocked with lidocaine with no epinephrine injections at 11 and 1 o'clock at the base of the penis. Then the infiltration is extended laterally to cover the entire circumference to the bottom of the shaft [51].

The penis is an extremity of the body (like the fingers, toes, and nose) so it is necessary to use the simple version of the anesthetic. Mixtures with epinephrine are not advisable because they cause contraction of the small arteries with subsequent tissue damage, including necrosis.

General anesthesia is chosen only for a small number of patients with severe anxiety or extreme intolerance to pain.

Selection of the soft tissue filler

* * *

The first step in selecting a soft tissue filler is deciding which product and which of its variants will be used for the procedure. As a general rule in the medical community, it is advisable to use only one type of soft tissue filler on the same area of the body. It is not a good idea to mix or superimpose different products in the same place and at the same time to prevent interactions or mixed results.

What is acceptable is to use different degrees of concentration or viscosity of the same product to achieve the desired increase in volume, which can be adjusted or transitioned to create an implant that is as natural as possible.

HA comes in different viscosity grades, and typically the heaviest one is used to achieve the best possible strength and longevity.

PCL has different versions based on its longevity (one, two, three, or four years). However, the injector and the patient usually decide to go with the longest-lasting version available on the local market.

PMMA is available in concentrations of 2%, 10%, and 30%. The former is very weak and is only used for minor volume changes or superficial facial wrinkles. In nonsurgical phalloplasty, only the two higher concentrations are used, either alone or in combination with each other. The typical approach for the circumcised patient is 30% in the proximal half of the shaft and 10% near the neck, so the implant gradually tapers as it approaches the glans. In the uncircumcised patient, it is recommended to only use the 10% concentration in moderate volume to avoid creating the "accordion effect" that's outlined in more detail in chapter 9.

Relaxed versus erect penis

Some physicians use intra-cavernosal injections to induce an erection before the placement of soft tissue filler. However, there is no proof of its benefit and is mostly a matter of preference and does not guarantee a better turnout.

Working with a relaxed or semi-erect penis seems to be more comfortable since the procedure requires extending, bending, twisting, and rotating the phallus to direct the micro cannula in all directions and reach the entire area of the prospective implant.

Another inconvenience of the induced erection method is that the swelling of the erectile organs creates pressure on the overlying structures, which temporarily limits the amount of room in the areolar space (the area of injection for the fillers).

Entry points and direction of implant

* * *

Some practices use a single entry point in the middle of the base of the penis and inject the soft tissue filler using a large cannula. Then they manually distribute the product through the shaft using their hands or surgical rollers.

More detail-oriented surgeons use several minor entry points and micro cannulas to reach every corner of the penile shaft, creating a smoother implant with less manipulation or massaging. The author's favorite technique is to drive the cannula in back and forth movements to deposit independent filler drops next to each other, covering the shaft's dorsum and sides.

The area that covers the urethra must remain free of soft tissue fillers because the corpus spongiosum is weak (even during erections), and fillers could compress the urethra and interfere with urination and ejaculation.

Micro cannulas

Small gauge micro cannulas are flexible and thin, with a small orifice on the side of the blunt tip. They facilitate a delicate approach to tissues and organs, like the penis, while protecting veins and arteries from being punctured.

Micro cannulas are the number one choice for the delicate and precise implant of injectable fillers in the penis.

Needles

The use of needles is almost ubiquitous even though we know that an accidental injection of soft tissue filler inside a vein or an artery can create severe side effects, such as embolism or necrosis, depending on the irrigation zone of the affected blood vessel.

Even physicians with extensive experience should refrain from using needles. Rounded-tip micro cannulas are the safest alternative because they offer almost complete protection against these accidents.

Injection gun

The injection gun gives more volume control when injecting the filler. Every time the injecting device is pulsed, the tissues receive a pre-established amount of product, around 1/100cc (varies according to the equipment used). This mechanical injection technique produces mini implants placed next to each other to create a uniform layer that is less prone to migration, clumping, and shifting.

Manual injections are just as good in the hands of experienced surgeons, and choosing one over the other is a matter of personal preference.

Massage during the procedure

* * *

The injection of soft tissue fillers is performed under simultaneous palpation and massaging or pressure rolling to ensure a uniform, thin coat implant.

The success of a phalloplasty procedure with soft tissue fillers depends on a synchronized effort between the injector and the patient. First, the physician performing the injections has to be skilled and use the extent of their expertise and knowledge to provide the best possible service. Second, it is equally necessary that the patient understands the instructions and performs the post-care tasks diligently, from follow-up visits to massage and the other essential recovery process steps.

At the end of the procedure and before leaving the treatment room, patients receive detailed, hands-on instructions on hygiene and manipulation and massage, as well as how to detect possible issues.

After the initial session, patients are scheduled to come back for follow-up visits to evaluate his skills at massaging the still-fresh implant and adherence to the post-care instructions.

Medical treatment

The most common medications prescribed to phalloplasty patients are:

* * *

- Anti-inflammatory drugs;
- Painkillers (even though most patients have only soreness);
- Antibiotics;
- Other specific prescription drugs that the patient may need.

Home-based procedures

Before their scheduled treatment, patients who have been stretching and pumping are encouraged to stop for at least one week before to allow any possible vascular damage to heal.

After the procedure, patients can stretch and pump as long as they don't hang more than 4-6 ounces or only create enough negative pressure to maintain the plastic capsule in place. The idea is to keep the penis slightly elongated, and the tissues expanded to a level that the pull or negative pressure doesn't create any pain.

A large number of patients ask about the benefits of oral supplements to enhance their production of collagen. Unfortunately, this is mostly a personal decision since there are no scientific studies that prove their benefit.

It is recommended that patients avoid self-prescribing medications (oral or topical) and always request a medical professional's opinion.

CHAPTER EIGHT
Post Care

The success of a girth enhancement procedure with soft tissue fillers ultimately depends on the parties involved: first the physician, then the patient. Since it takes time for the soft tissue filler to stabilize and establish itself in the tissues, most post-procedure care is in the patient's hands.

Physicians must concentrate on doing their best, as it should be in any medical procedure. The patient should then strictly adhere to the follow-up indications that they receive after the treatment.

Post-care instructions vary greatly depending on the soft tissue filler used and the medical practice's standards, so patients should understand and inquire about every detail that they can think of before engaging in the post-care treatment on their own.

The medical practice should provide detailed instruction and information about:

Swelling, bruising

Some patients develop inflammation and bruising that can be severe, especially if the injector is very aggressive.

Under normal conditions there is no pain after a girth enhancement procedure; if anything, there will be minimal soreness, more noticeable to the touch and mainly when pressure is applied. Patients do not need to take medication for this, as both swelling and bruising disappear in less than 72 hours.

The first night after the procedure

The first night after the procedure is the most difficult of all. The patient should sleep naked and interrupt his sleep to massage himself once or twice during the night. He will be able to sleep on his back or sides, even on his stomach, but taking care not to put any kind of pressure on the penis, which must remain free and without kinks. Stretchers and pumps are not used while sleeping.

In our practice, we ask the patient to remain in town overnight and return for supervision the following morning so that the doctor can assess his post-care acumen in case he needs more instruction.

Clothing

Patients should wear loose clothes that can be easily removed without hurting the treated area: shorts or sweat pants with elastic waistbands and boxers. Avoid the use of lycra, tight underwear, jeans, and similar restrictive garments.

Hygiene

It is recommended to take a bath before the procedure. Avoid using moisturizers, powders, and perfumes, especially in the genital area. Showers are permitted immediately after the procedure; however, the patient must wash his hands thoroughly before washing the penis. If the entry points are still open, the patient is instructed to use plenty of soap, rinse, and tap-dry the area. No soaking; the use of swimming pools, saunas, or jacuzzis should be avoided for one week.

Sexual intercourse

Sexual intercourse should be reestablished gradually and carefully. The most critical period with microsphere implants (PCL and PMMA) is during the first 10 days when the vehicle is absorbed and tissue ingrowth begins. Then, as the implant establishes itself by growing new collagen, it will become more stable and the patient will be able to return to everyday life. Ideally, patients should avoid sexual intercourse or vigorous masturbation for four weeks.

Since HA is more unstable, it requires more care and a longer period of sexual abstinence to allow the thin capsule to form and obtain some firmness. Ideally, these patients should avoid sexual intercourse or vigorous masturbation for six weeks, as well as tight gripping of the penis for a longer period of time. Reportedly, patients with high HA doses can leave finger pressure marks on their penis after a high-pressure grip.

Erections and gently erotic manipulation are allowed at any time, as long as it is done under highly hygienic conditions using disinfectant gels and / or condoms, and avoiding contact with body fluids and penetration.

Post-treatment massaging

Extreme hygiene and proper massage are the primary responsibility of the patient, since both aftercare requirements extend for several days after the procedure.

The required massage varies significantly between medical practices and also between the different products used for phalloplasty.

HA patients need a firm massage. With the penis between their palms, they need to roll it like forming a play dough cylinder. HA remains a gel and can be easily moved, so it is also recommended to maintain a compressive bandage for four weeks or longer. The firmness of the compressive dressing should be strong enough to keep the shape of the body of the penis but not too tight that it interferes with blood flow.

Patients who receive a microsphere-based implant (PMMA

or PCL) require a systematic, dedicated, and cautious massage to avoid product agglomerations and reduce the possibility of irregularities. It is helpful to stretch, bend, or support the penis with one hand while the other one palpates and dissipates potential clumps.

This massage is essential, and patients must receive hands-on training or continuous supervision before they are released. Patients must make an effort and concentrate during the first phase of the massage, where the goal is to palpate the implant. Next, they should apply gentle pressure with the fingertips and feel the implant to locate irregularities, such as product clumping or empty areas.

Once the nodules are located, pinch with two fingers pressing firmly, or use a plastic or metal roller, and push the excess product in opposite directions so that excessive accumulations are smoothed out and voids are filled in. Typically, sliding will be from the entry point in all directions towards the periphery or towards the periphery or a specific area if it shows a lack of product. The roller will be rotated slowly, turning little by little and maintaining firm pressure, but not so much pressure that it could damage the tissue. If the soft tissue filler is oozing, pinch the entry point area with two fingers while it is still open, as this prevents the product from forming a tiny superficial nodule that later looks like a small pearl embedded in the skin.

* * *

Careless palpation or blind massage does not help to soften up the implant and may, in fact, damage it.

The massage should be done for 10-15 minutes and repeated every 6 hours for the first week, then once a day, at noon, for four weeks for PCL & PMMA patients or for six weeks for patients that received HA. Massaging and pressing are primarily helpful during the first 72 hours but becomes less impactful by the end of the first week as the carrier absorbs. Massaging should stop by the end of the first week when tissue ingrowth starts.

Erections do not adversely affect the massage; instead, they facilitate the process to the point that it is actually better to induce them during the recovery time using erection stimulants like tadalafil, 5 mg. daily. This regimen also results in a partially erected penis, which helps prevent retraction during rest.

Stretching and pumping

A possible complication that some patients may experience after the procedure is caused by penile retraction. Therefore, it is crucial to keep the penis relaxed and, if possible, semi-erect because retraction (especially if it is severe) can cause a formation of rings or "accordions."

Some medications help keep the penis relaxed, such as low-dose tadalafil and tamsulosin, so they should be prescribed and explained by the treating physician.

As part of the treatments at home, it is advisable to keep the genital area warm by wearing comfortable and protective underwear. It's also important to keep stress to a minimum and take time to relax for at least a week. The use of stretchers and pumps is recommended to limit retraction.

Stretchers

A wide variety of stretchers are available and patients are free to choose the most comfortable one. Although it is recommended to select one that attaches in areas free of soft tissue fillers, such as in the space directly behind the glans at one end and at the pelvic area at the other.

Patients are instructed to use the minimum weight necessary to keep the penis comfortably stretched. It is important to bear in mind that the goal is to keep the penis comfortably elongated during the recovery period.

* * *

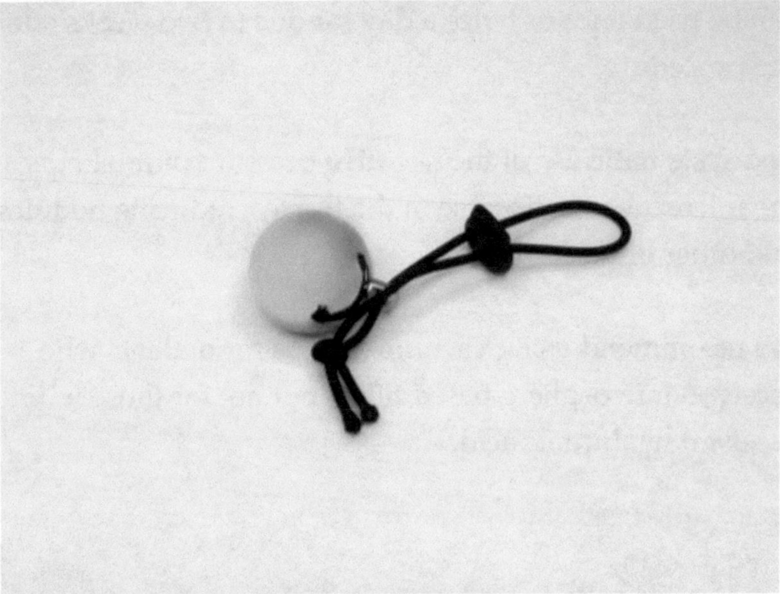

Figure 8.1. The basic stretcher attaches to the neck of the penis.

The stretcher should be used immediately after the procedure and for as long as possible during the day.

Pumps

There is also a wide variety of vacuum pumps available, ranging from a simple bulb to sophisticated products with pressure gauges and other attachments that are not required for phalloplasty purposes.

What is needed is a basic model with a suitable size for the new dimensions of the penis. It is recommended to apply moderate negative pressure that's sufficient to keep the bulb in place. It will be left on for five to ten minutes and can be used once or twice a day for one to two weeks after the procedure.

The systematic use of the negative pressure pump helps the microspheres disperse in the tissues, reducing nodules and other imperfections.

We recommend using vacuum pumps for patients who received microsphere-based fillers but not for those who received hyaluronic acid.

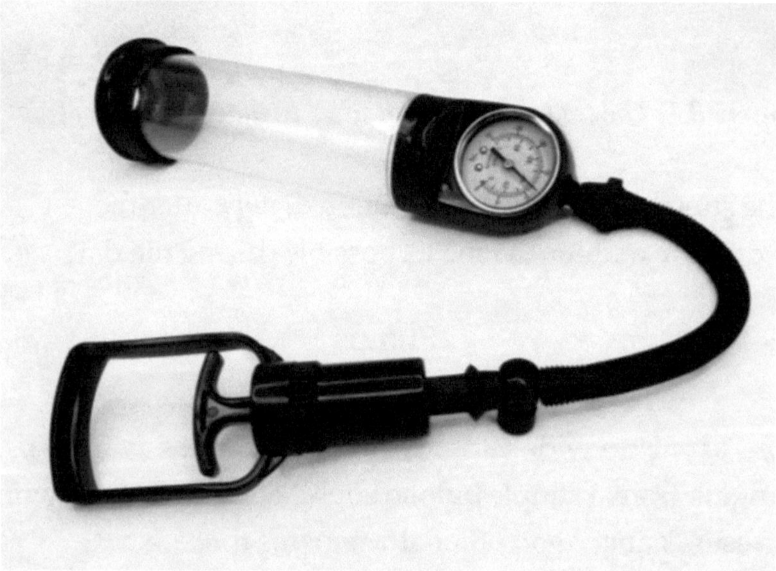

Figure 8.2. Simple design pump with no bells and whistles.

Wrapping

PMMA and PCL implants are unstable for around 10 days; HA for much longer. During this time, it is advisable to use a compression bandage (from the base to the neck of the penis) that maintains the smooth and cylindrical shape of the shaft. There are different compression bandages, such as silicone sleeves, self-adherent elastic bandages, and tubular bandages like Tubigrip®. The author recommends the self-adherent dressing because it is easier to adjust its pressure at any time.

The pressure of the bandage must be firm enough to maintain the shape of the penis but not so intense that it interferes with its blood flow. The dressing should be relaxed or removed if the patient feels discomfort, pain, or the glans looks abnormally white or blue.

It is recommended to use the compressive bandage during the day for four weeks in patients receiving PCL or PMMA and six or more weeks in those receiving HA.

Medications and supplements

Regardless of the tamsulosin and tadalafil recommendations mentioned previously, phalloplasty patients only need antibiotics in some cases, depending on the doctor's judgment. This also applies to the occasional use of pain relievers and anti-inflammatories. In addition, we have no evidence to suggest that the use of growth hormone or testosterone promotes the formation of more or better collagen.

* * *

Certain medications that affect collagen, such as non-steroidal anti-inflammatory drugs (ibuprofen, naproxen, and the like), anti-rheumatics, and others, could interfere with new collagen formation. Still, it is the patient's responsibility to consult with their doctor for authorization to temporarily interrupt their treatment.

As a general rule, patients should refrain from self-medicating, whether they are topical products (such as antibiotics or steroid creams), oral, or injectable medications. Also, there is no scientific evidence that supplements affect the results of nonsurgical phalloplasty.

CHAPTER NINE
Limitations and Complications

Limitations

There is no perfect technique for penile girth enhancement. Still, injectable implants are currently among the safest and most natural ways to augment the penis's volume while keeping its natural shape and aesthetics.

Like all medical-cosmetic procedures, nonsurgical phalloplasty has certain limitations. Therefore, it is always important to keep in mind that moderation should prevail. The physician should guide the patient, keeping in mind that it is not worth taking any high risk in an elective procedure like this.

Lack of circumcision is a limitation but not necessarily a contraindication. Uncircumcised patients may be good candidates, but their approach must be cautious and moderate, and it is recommended to use low volume and (when available) products with lesser concentrations. Using high volumes in these patients can cause the "accordion effect" defect and other significant irregularities.

The size and shape of the penis are also essential considerations: the smaller the penis, the more difficult it will be to achieve an acceptable cosmetic increase. Some shapes (missile, inverse truncated cone) have a greater degree of difficulty in attaining homogeneous growth. While patients with small, pointed glans are also limited as to the amount of soft tissue filler that can be used, as increasing the volume of the shaft of this type of penis can make the glans look disproportionately tiny.

Unfortunately, nonsurgical phalloplasty does not offer any advantage to patients with micropenis.

Patients with thin and loose skin (uncircumcised or with a loose circumcision) are also tricky to manage since the soft tissue filler can migrate through the shaft, causing irregularities. Thin, sagging skin is more common in fair-skinned, elderly, and uncircumcised patients.

Some patients present fibrotic rings at the circumcision scar or at other levels of the shaft of the penis. These rings can cause skin constriction and tissue displacement; however, they are not noticeable in all patients. Sometimes they only appear as the soft tissue filler is applied. Annular depressions caused by fibrous rings are not generally a big deal, typically requiring only a touch-up session to precisely repair the area.

Complications

While complications are rare, they can happen even under

the best care and at the hands of the most skilled surgeons and dedicated patients.

We can divide the penile girth enhancement complications into three main groups:

- Technique-related complications can arise independently of the soft tissue filler used, but safe methods and the injectors' experience reduce them substantially. This group of complications includes excessive pain due to incomplete anesthesia, necrosis due to accidental injection of the filler into an artery or vein, infection due to inadequate sterilization, bruising, bleeding, and inflammation.

- Product-related complications can occur when the substance or substances injected interact negatively with the body's natural tissues. Products containing bovine collagen or other biologic materials can trigger allergic reactions. The host's immune response can create granulomas, and some absorbable fillers can leave residual fibrosis.

- Host-related complications are due to inadequate home post-care and can come from excessive or premature manipulation or intercourse, lousy hygiene (either deficient or exaggerated), and other similar factors. Among the most common are infections, dislocation of the implant, and contact dermatitis.

* * *

The three groups of complications described above can appear and disappear quickly (acute) or be insidious (chronic).

Acute Complications

Redness, bruising, inflammation, and soreness happen in most patients. This condition varies widely in intensity, but under normal circumstances they resolve in around 72 hours.

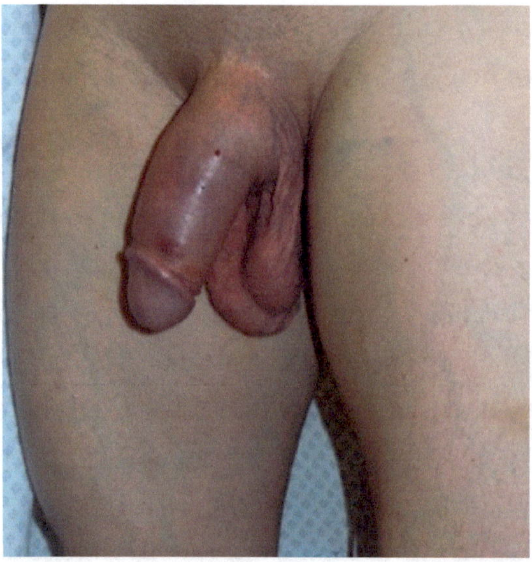

Figure 9.1. Bruising and inflammation.

Necrosis or local tissue death is a severe acute problem that can create permanent damage, like scarring, retraction, and deformity. It is a technique-related complication due to accidental deposits of filler into an artery that blocks its blood flow with subsequent damage. The artery blockage is an accident that can happen with any soft tissue filler or even fat transfer. The use of rounded tip micro cannulas as an alternative for sharp needles minimizes this possibility.

Fournier's gangrene is a severe complication that can come after infections in the area of the genitals. It happens mostly in older male individuals with co-existing conditions like diabetes, cirrhosis, chemotherapy, HIV infection, etc. However, Fournier's gangrene has not been reported after penile implants or injections of soft tissue fillers.

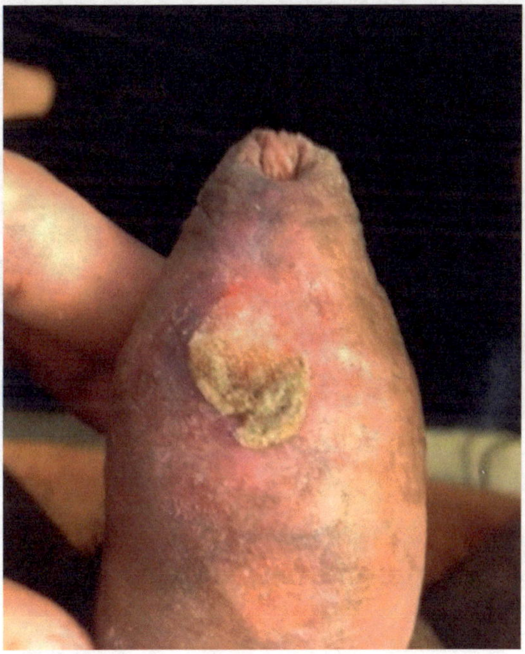

Figure 9.2. Necrosis.

* * *

Infection is a rare complication that can be related to a precarious injection technique or inadequate patient care. The presence of microspheres in the soft tissue filler triggers the host's cellular immune response. The immediate arrival of phagocytes that control bacterial growth usually contains infections in their early stage. Gel-based fillers may offer less immune protection, but it's often enough to prevent this complication.

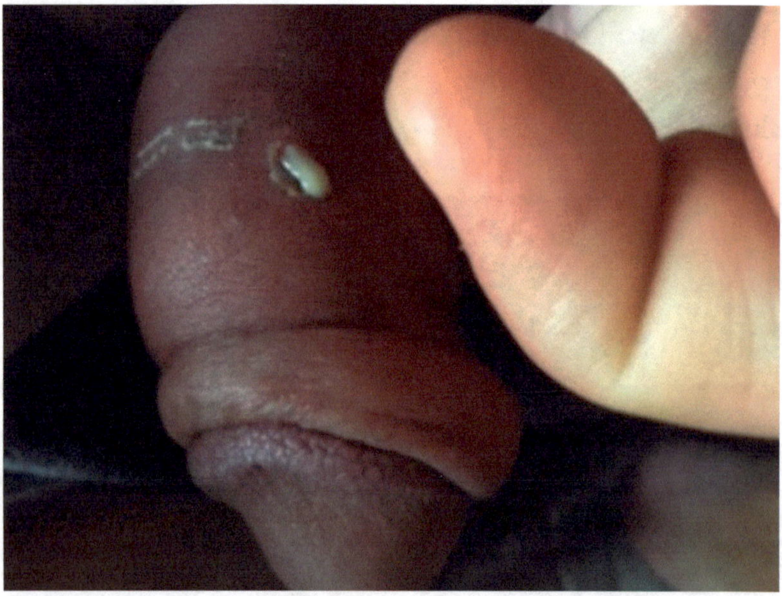

Figure 9.3. Acute infection.

Chronic and Late Complications

Most long-term complications are associated with the shape and volume of the implant: overcorrection, nodules, voids, and asymmetry.

The "pig in a blanket" effect is a common complication in overcorrected circumcised individuals, especially in the presence of loose or partial circumcision. The only way to avoid it is by limiting the filler volume, taper from the center to the neck, and lower product concentrations when possible. This effect is more notorious in the relaxed penis, but most patients don't mind it because their penis looks good when erect.

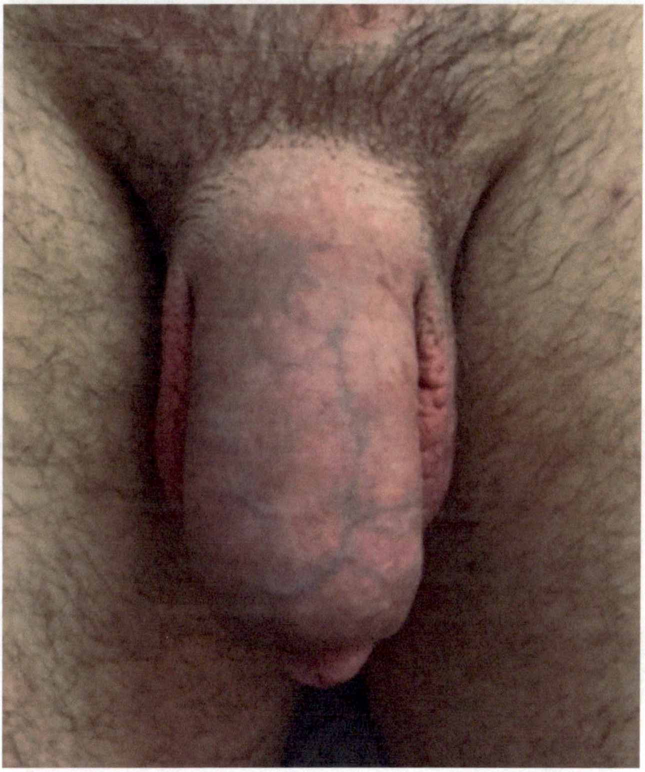

Figure 9.4. Pig in a blanket effect.

* * *

The "accordion effect" is an inevitable complication in uncircumcised individuals. When the patient pulls the skin backward, it moves along with the implant and creates an unsightly bulge at the base of the penis. It that can be big enough to interfere with penetration in some patients.

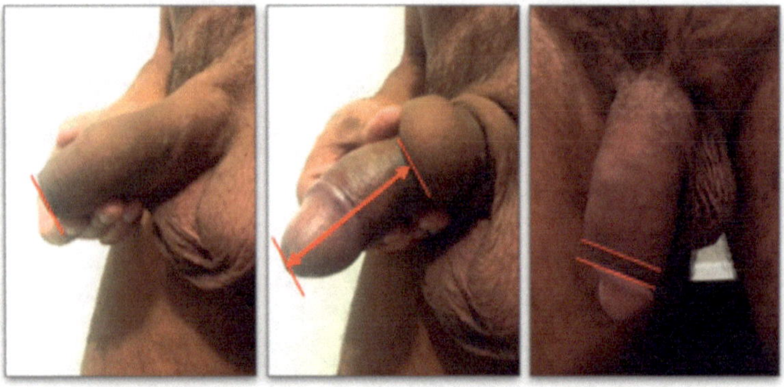

Figure 9.5. Accordion effect showing its correction after circumcision.

The figure above shows a patient that had two sessions of PMMA 10%. It looked reasonable at first glance (left), but when retracting the skin (center) the fold created by the implant was big and interfered with intercourse. The third image (right) shows the same patient after his circumcision and a touch-up session with the same filler. The red lines demonstrate the mobility of the skin before and after the surgical correction.

Nodules and voids: Imperfections like nodules and depressions are common complications after the implant of soft tissue fillers. Patients should expect some degree of flaws that can appear within weeks after their treatment.

• Imperfections associated with hyaluronic acid can be reversed with hyaluronidase injections, an enzyme that will dissolve the product.

• Flaws after calcium hydroxylapatite or polycaprolactone (Radiesse®, Ellansé®) will diminish over time as the implant is slowly absorbed.

• Imperfections after PMMA will be permanent unless corrected with touch-up sessions or surgical extraction.

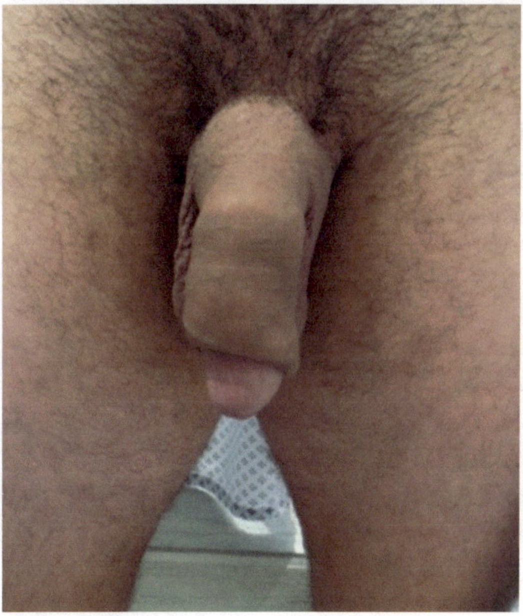

Figure 9.6. Nodules and voids.

* * *

Cysts: Soft tissue fillers should be deposited as a thin layer that "organizes" with collagen growing from the injected material's external and internal surfaces. Injecting an excess of soft tissue filler prevents the collagen growth from reaching the center of the implant, leaving a core of unprocessed product that turns into a cyst (a semi-hard lump with a viscous liquid core).

Cysts are poorly tolerated. The blood vessels cannot grow into it, and they are prone to infection, spontaneous opening, and draining.

Preventing the formation of cysts requires the patient to come back for multiple sessions of thin layers of fillers, so one organizes before implanting the next one.

The typical time between sessions is 6 weeks for microsphere-based implants, and timing is more flexible for hyaluronic acid patients.

* * *

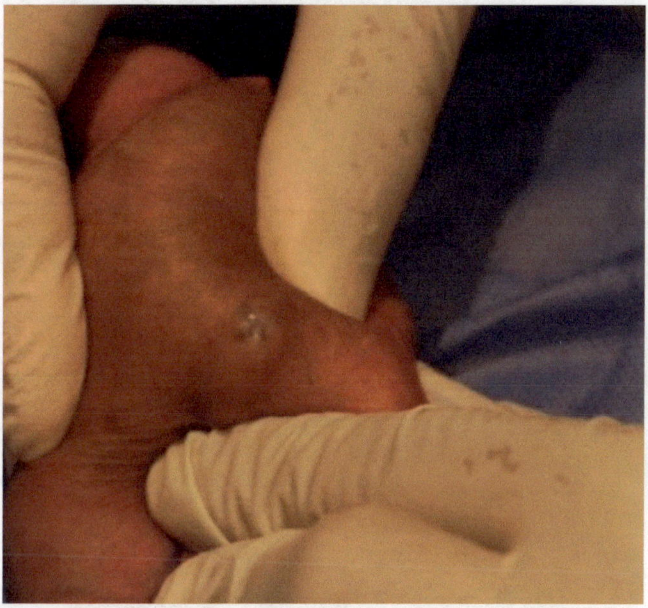

Figure 9.7. Cyst.

Asymmetry is mostly a technique-related complication resulting from depositing more material on one side or filler's migration. It can be corrected with touch-up sessions.

* * *

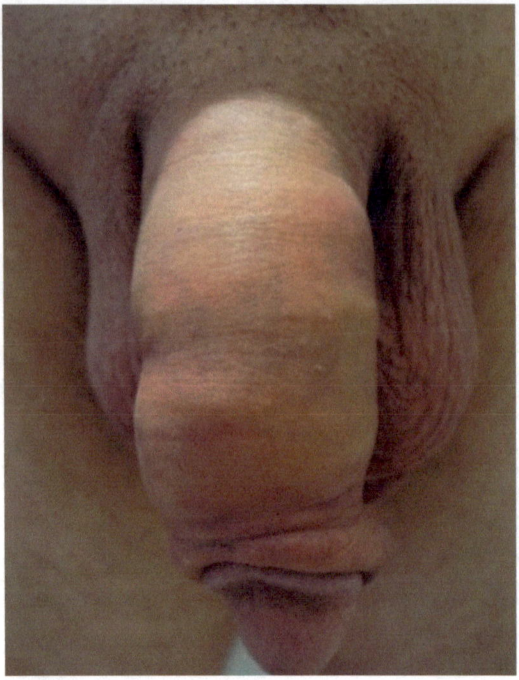

Figure 9.8. Asymmetry.

Granulomas: Foreign body granulomas can occur with all injectable fillers. They have to be distinguished from nodules, as they may look the same but are much different.

Granulomas are active lesions that usually appear after several months, even years. The reaction happens in all injected sites that show clear signs of inflammation, redness, tenderness, higher temperature, and pain [52, 53].

Diagnosing and treating granulomas at an early stage will solve them within a few weeks. The treatment of choice for this reaction includes cortisone or other anti-inflammatory drugs. Reportedly, some laser treatments also help, but surgery is not recommended. They may also resolve spontaneously without treatment.

Active granulomas are not typical and can be confused with inactive nodules. The author has not witnessed any cases of true granuloma in the penis. Since most reports do not differentiate nodules from granulomas, no specific instances have been found in the literature.

The following table summarizes the differences between a nodule and a granuloma:

Condition	Nodule	Granuloma
Can appear immediately after the injection of the soft tissue filler	Yes	No
Appears on previously soft, flat skin, weeks or months after the injections	No	Yes
Shows signs of acute, active inflammatory reaction (swelling, pain, heat)	No	Yes
Immune-mediated allergic reaction	No	Yes
Affects isolated areas of the implant / single or several asymmetric lesions	Yes	No
Affects all areas of the implant, even if it was done in different areas of the body	No	Yes
Redness, itch, inflammation, heat, local pain	No	Yes
Responds to steroid (cortisone) injection	Poorly	Yes
Easy surgical extraction	Yes	No
Can disappear spontaneously	No	Yes

Table 9.1. Differences between nodule and granuloma.

Multi-treated patients

* * *

For some patients, enlarging their penis turns into an obsession. Some ask for results that are not achievable and insist on additional procedures against their doctor's best advice. Unfortunately, these patients will often find someone willing to take them, even when they have scars, deformities, and other signs of over manipulation and abuse. They are a challenging group of individuals who can barely wait to recover before jumping into the next procedure, even after severe complications and deformity.

Multiple surgical incisions and scars are very damaging to the penis: they leave marks, fibrosis, deformity, retraction, and sometimes ulceration, which opens another vicious cycle. Multi-treated patients are high risk, and they are not good candidates for nonsurgical phalloplasty.

* * *

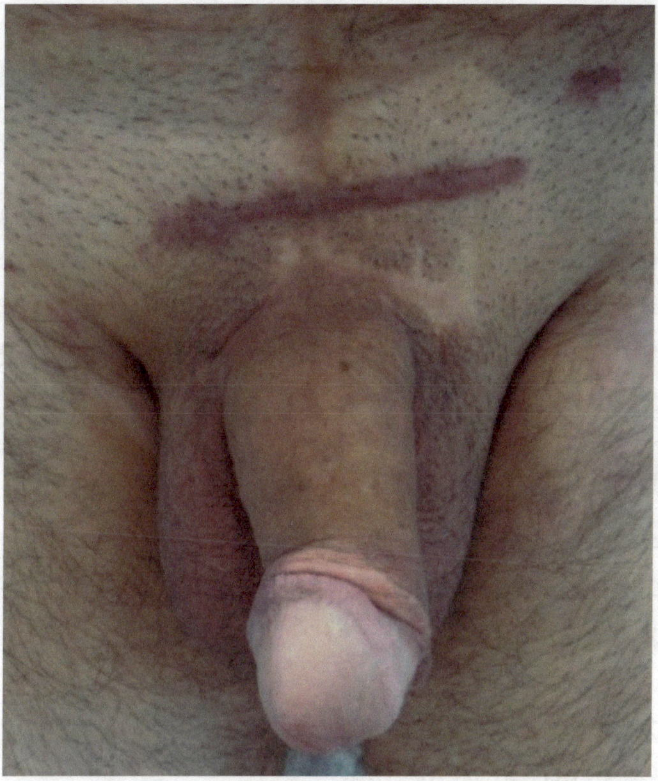

Figure 9.9. Multi-treated patient.

Discussion

One extensive study of 729 patients that underwent phalloplasty with PMMA [7] showed the following results:

- Postoperative swelling and internal inflammation resolved within a few days.

- Sterile exudate through the entry points is a common occurrence that resolves in approximately 24 hours.

* * *

• Urinary symptoms were not present because the implant did not cover the urethral part of the spongy body.

• More than half of the patients (52%) reported minimum to severe irregularities, such as single nodules, multiple nodules, rugged ridges, micro-nodules at the entry points, indentations, or voids. However, 87% were satisfied with their results.

• Twenty-two percent of the patients who reported irregularities were non-circumcised, and their penile skin was more relaxed and loose, contributing to their outcomes.

• A small number of patients (0.4%) needed surgical removal of one or more nodules.

• Inactive nodules were often confused with granulomas by patients and some physicians, but we could not document any valid instances of "true granulomas."

• There was no PMMA translocation or migration to neighboring areas.

• Patient satisfaction was measured on a scale of 1 (very dissatisfied) to 10 (extremely satisfied). Overall satisfaction with the procedure was 8.7, a very similar statistical number as with surgical facelifts.

* * *

The correction of most irregularities is possible through meticulous smoothening with micro-drops of the same filler. Surgical partial or complete removal should be the last option.

CHAPTER TEN

Anecdotes

Every patient is a story of their own. Phalloplasty is a procedure that involves the patient and his sexual partner; it is an elective procedure that could compare to breast implants. However, it still has very little support from both physicians and the public, and it is as controversial — or even more so — as large tattoos or other extreme body modifications.

Some patients educate themselves on the technique and the product, while others take it lightly. It doesn't surprise that the latter is more prone to choosing the wrong product or a bad injector.

The following are only a few instances of daily episodes seen in patients undergoing phalloplasty:

What I'm doing here?

It is not unusual to hear patients coming out of the dressing room, all ready to start the process, and expressing their last-minute concern about something. They giggle and quietly say, "I don't know what I'm doing here!" It is a sign that they need to be reassured that they are in good hands and, most importantly, that there is still time to call back the procedure. It is a critical moment when they need time to take a breath. If the anxiety escalates and the patient becomes more excited about the treatment, the best alternative is to postpone the procedure.

The unhappy wife

Talking to a patient after his first "dick enlargement" procedure, he revealed that he wanted to surprise his wife, hoping to spice up their relationship in celebration of their twenty-fifth anniversary. He alleged that since she had breast implants, he was entitled to have his own enlargement. First, he saw my facial expression, and then I saw his... Unfortunately, my suspicions were correct: the wife hated that he planned everything behind her back, and she firmly stated that she did not need any more girth from her husband. She told him something to the effect of, "Yes, I got boob implants, but I don't put them inside your body." The last I knew, she was considering a divorce.

Messy financials

A patient came for his third round and declared that he was going through tough financial times. We recommended calling off his session, but he insisted. Weeks later, he wrote a bitter email claiming that he couldn't put together the down payment for his house and blamed it on the girth enhancement treatment cost.

Psychologically unstable

This patient went through his first procedure with no outstanding issues: he was excited and cooperative and didn't show any behavioral problems. He went home happy, but the very next day he claimed that the implant had migrated to his heart. He was very anxious, had palpitations, and decided to go to a cardiologist to find out that … nothing was wrong. The following day he claimed the implant had migrated to his stomach and needed a gastroenterologist to assure him that he was okay. The migration drama continued, and at some point he told me that he was such a wreck that his girlfriend had to slap him in the face a couple of times. By the end of the first week he ended up in a local urology practice for surgical removal of his wicked implant.

Greed

A surgeon called me to perform a girth enhancement implant with soft tissue fillers on a patient with his suspensory ligament cut. After his recovery, he had three more sessions of injectable fillers with the excuse that his wife was loose after two babies. After his third treatment I told him that his gains were extreme and that I didn't recommend any more procedures. However, he went back to his surgeon and persuaded him to do many more sessions (I suspect more than a dozen).

His penis ended up gigantic, and one day he came back to me feeling miserable because he had subsequently divorced and then found it tough to find a mate because of his enormous penis. So he had the implant surgically removed but, to my dismay, showed up months later and disclosed that he missed his girth and wanted to restart the process.

Undisclosed conditions

To avoid rejecting patients, especially when they travel from afar, we have them respond to an online questionnaire. For example, one patient reported that he didn't know the size of his penis but established that he wanted an increase of one inch in his girth, failing to disclose that he had a micropenis. As a result, he traveled across Europe, the Atlantic Ocean, and the continental US for his treatment.

It was disappointing for both of us when I discovered his condition and told him that I wouldn't advise more than a 0.25-inch increase to maintain harmony.

Undisclosed previous procedures

This patient from the East Coast had his first session with us and disappeared for a couple of years. He came back for what we thought was his second session, but while exploring him I found out that he had gone for two more procedures with a known charlatan that uses large doses of silicone oil, presenting it as PMMA. We rejected the patient, who lost considerable time and money.

Phallocentrism

One patient came for his first procedure, and even though he had a good evolution and results he went through tough times worrying about possible consequences and other imaginary possibilities to the point that his physician refused to take him for a second procedure.

Several months later, he called again requesting to speak to the doctor, explained several reasons why he had reacted so bad in the past, and promised that he would refrain from doing it again.

He told the doctor that his life and future happiness depended entirely on having a big, perfect penis, which is typical for patients with phallogocentrism. No need to wonder; he got the same response again: "Phalloplasty is not for you."

Encountered feelings

One patient showed up with his upset wife. She was unhappy, unwilling to communicate, and constantly arguing with him because he was doing the procedure against her will. The treating physicians left them alone so that they could come to an agreement before proceeding. After very long deliberation, she reluctantly accepted and barely supported his decision to go for his phalloplasty procedure. She stayed in the waiting room, still complaining until the end of the husband's treatment. About two months later, our patient coordinator got a request for a second session for this patient. To our surprise, it turned out that it was the wife generating the phone call. Well, I guess we're all entitled to change our minds, aren't we?

BIBLIOGRAPHY

1. Kelley JH, Eraklis AJ . A procedure for lengthening the phallus in boys with exstrophy of the bladder. J Pediatr Surg 1971; 6: 645–649.

2. Khawaja HA. Complications of fat transfer. In: Shiffman M. Autologous Fat Transfer. Springer, Berlin, Heidelberg. 2010.

3. Alter G, Salgado C, Chim H. Aesthetic surgery of the male genitalia. Semin Plast Surg 2011; 25: 189-195.

4. Krakovsky A. Up-to-date surgical techniques for penile augmentation with AlloDerm. Am J Cosm Surg. 2008;25(3):135-44.

5. Xu T, Bai W, Li Q et al. Complications and management of penile girth enhancement with acellular dermal matrix. J Sex Med 2019;16(12):2011-17.

6. Keefe J, Wauk L, Chu S, DeLustro F. Clinical use of injectable bovine collagen: A decade of experience. Clin Mater. 1992;9(3-4):155-162.

7. Casavantes L, Morales P, Lemperle G. Penile girth enhancement with PMMA-based soft tissue fillers. J Sex Med 2016;13:1414-1422.

8. Bigelow J. The development of circumcision in Judaism. In: Bigelow J., The joy of uncircumcising. Hourglass Book Publishing, Aptos, California 95001, 1992, 1995.

9. Hodges F. The ideal prepuce in ancient Greece and Rome: Male genital aesthetics and their relation to lipodermos, circumcision, foreskin restoration, and the kynodesme. The Bulletin of the History of Medicine. 2001;75(3):375-405.

10. Veale D. Miles S, Bramley S, et al. Am I normal? A systematic review and construction of nomograms for flaccid and erect penis length and circumference in up to 15521 men. BJU Int. 2015;115(6):978-86.

11. Francken A, van de Wiel H, et al. What importance do women attribute to the size of the penis? Eur Urol. 2002;42(5):426-31.

12. Wylie K, Eardley I. Penile size and the 'Small Penis Syndrome.' BJU Int. 2007;99(6):1449-55.

13. Lever J, Frederick D, Peplau L. Does size matter? Men's and women's views on penis size across the lifespan. Psych Men Masc 2006;7(3)129-143.

14. Prause N, Park J, Leung S, Miller G. Women's preferences for penis size: A new research method using selection among 3D models. PLOS One. 2015;10(9).

15. Payne K, Thaler L, et al. Sensation and sexual arousal in circumcised and uncircumcised men. J Sex Med. 2007;4(3): 667–674.

16. Laumann E, Masi C, Zuckerman E. Circumcision in the United States: Prevalence, Prophylactic Effects, and Sexual Practice. JAMA. 1997;277(13):1052-57.

17. Callens N, De Cuypere G, Van Hoecke E, et al. Sexual quality of life after hormonal and surgical treatment, including phalloplasty, in men with micropenis:

A review. J Sex Med 2013;10(12):2890-903.

18. Tang S, Kamat D, Santucci R. Modern Management of Adult-acquired Buried Penis. Urology 2008;72(1):124-7.

19. Pryor J, Akkus E, Alter G, et al. Peyronie's Disease. J Sex Med. 2004;1(1):110-116.

20. Carrion R. Ventral Phalloplasty. J Sex Med 2010;7(9):2914-17.

21. Veale D, Miles S, Read J, et al. Penile Dysmorphic Disorder: Development of a Screening Scale. Archives of Sexual Behavior. 2015;44(8):2311-2321.

22. Murtagh J. The 'Small' Penis Syndrome. Australian Family Physician. 1989;18(3):218-220.

23. Khawaja H, Hernandez-Perez E. Fat transfer review: Controversies, complications, their prevention, and treatment. Int J Cosm Surg Best Derm. 2004;4(2).

24. Kawaja H, Shiffman M. Penile Enhancement. In: Shiffman M., Di Giusseppe A. (eds) Cosmetic Surgery. Springer, Berlin, Heidelberg. 2013.

25. Vardi Y, Har-Shai Y, Gil T, Gruenwald I. A critical analysis of penile enhancement procedures for patients with normal penile size: surgical techniques, success, and complications. Eur Urol. 2008; 54(5):1042-50.

26. Jung G. Penile Girth Enhancement with Allograft. In: Park N., Kim S., Moon D. (eds) Penile Augmentation. Springer, Berlin, Heidelgerg. 2016.

27. Shirvanian V, Lemperle G, Araujo Pinto C, Elist J. Shortened penis post penile prosthesis implantation treated with subcutaneous soft silicone penile implant: Case report. Int J Impot Res. 2014;26(3):100-4.

28. Austoni E, Colombo F, Romano A, et al. Soft prosthesis implant and relaxing albugineal incision with saphenous grafting for surgical therapy of Peyronie's Disease: A 5-year Experience and long-term follow-up on 145 operated patients. Eur. Urol. 2005;47(2):223-9.

29. Alter G. Penile enlargement surgery. Techniques in Urology. 1998;4(2):70-6.

30. Chen Y, Ji C, Wu B, et al. Application of MEDPOR Surgical Implant in Modified Penile Elongation: Review of 19 Cases. Ann Plast Surg. 2017;78(5)549-551.

31. Li C, Kayes O, Kell P, et al. Penile suspensory ligament division for penile augmentation: indications and results. Eur Urol. 2006;49(4):729-33.

32. Figler B, Chery L, Friedrich J, et al. Limited Panniculectomy for Adult Buried Penis Repair. Plast Reconstr Surg. 2015;136(5):1090-2.

33. Caso J, Keating M, Miranda-Sousa A, Carrion R. Ventral Phalloplasty. Asian J Androl. 2008;10(1):155-57.

34. Kim J, Kwak T, Jeon B, et al. Human glans penis augmentation using injectable hyaluronic acid gel. Int J Impot Res. 2003;15:439-43.

35. Yang D, Ko K, Lee S, et al. Efficacy and safety of newly developed cross-linked dextran gel injection for glans penis augmentation with a novel technique. Asian J Androl. 2018;20(1):80-4.

36. Bodiwala D, Summerton D, Terry T. Testicular Prosthesis: Development and Modern Usage. Ann R Coll Surg Engl 2007;(89)4:349-53.

37. Schultheiss D, Truss M, Stief C, et al.

Uncircumcision: A Historical Review of Preputial Restoration. Plas Rec Surg. 1998;101(7).

38. Kwak T, Oh M, Kim J, Moon D. The effects of penile girth enhancement using injectable hyaluronic acid gel, a filler. J Sex Med. 2011;8(12):3407-3413.

39. Lemperle G, de Fazio S, Nicolau P. ArteFill: A third-generation permanent dermal filler and tissue stimulator. Clin Plast Surg. 2006;33(4):551-65.

40. Lemperle G, Morhenn V, Charrier U. Human histology and persistence of various injectable filler substances for soft tissue augmentation. Aesthetic Plastic Surgery. 2003;27(5):356-66.

41. Kim J, Van Arbel D. Neocollagenesis in human tissue injected with a polycaprolactone-based dermal filler. Journal of Cosmetic and Laser Therapy. 2015;17:99-101.

42. Jansen D, Graivier M. Evaluation of a Calcium-hydroxylapatite-based Implant (Radiesse) for Facial soft-tissue Augmentation. Plastic and Reconstructive Surgery 2006;118(3):22S-30S.

43. Narins R, Beer K. Liquid injectable silicone: A review of its history, immunology, technical considerations, complications and potential. Plast Reconstr Surg. 2006; 118(3):77S-84S.

44. Jones D, Carruthers A, Orentreich D, et al. Highly purified 1000-cSt silicone oil for treatment of human immunodeficiency virus-associated facial lipoatrophy: An open pilot trial. Dermatol Surg 2004;30(10): 1279-86.

45. Yacobi Y, Tsivian A, Grinberg R, Kessler O. Short-term results of incremental penile girth enhancement using

liquid injectable silicone: Words of praise for a change. Asian J Androl 2007;9:408–13.

46. Barnett J, Barnett C. Treatment of Acne Scars with Liquid Silicone Injections: 30- year Perspective. Dermatol Surg. 2006;31(4):1542-9.

47. Sharp G, Oates J. Nonsurgical medical penile girth augmentation: A retrospective study of psychological and psychosexual outcomes. Aesthetic Surgery Journal. 2018;39(3):306-16.

48. Veale D, Eshkeveri E, Read J, et al. Beliefs about penis size: Validation of a scale for men ashamed about their penis size. J Sex Med. 2014;11(1):84-92.

49. Gelbard M, Dorey F, James K. The Natural History of Peyronie's Disease. The Journal of Urology. 1990;144(6):1376-9.

50. Lemperle G, Casavantes L. Penis enlargement by injecting PMMA microspheres. Aesthetic Surgery. 2018;XK-4b:1-11.

51. Malkoc E, Ates F, Uguz S, et al. Effective Penile block for circumcision in adults. Wien Klin Wochenschr. 2012;124(13-14):434-8.

52. Lemperle G, Gauthier-Hazan N, Wolters M, et al. Foreign Body Granulomas after all Injectable Dermal Fillers. Part 1. Possible Causes. Plast Reconstr Surg 2009;123(6):1842-63.

53. Lee J, Kim Y. Foreign Body Granulomas after the use of Dermal Fillers: Pathophysiology, Clinical Appearance, Histologic Features, and Treatment. Arch Plast Surg. 2015;42(2):232-9.

54. Lemperle G, Bauthier-Hazan N. Foreign body granulomas after all injectable dermal fillers: Part 2. Treatment Options. Plast Reconstr Surg. 2009;123(6):1864-73.

Made in the USA
Monee, IL
05 November 2026

67806826R00085